THE
PALEO
MIRACLE:
50 Real Stories of
Health Transformation

compiled and edited by

Joseph Salama and Christina Lianos

ISBN-13: 978-1480286344
ISBN-10: 1480286346

This book is dedicated to my perfect children Amira and Mark and to the brilliant, talented, and gorgeous Eve Haapala (page 84) who was paleo before it was called paleo, and whom I would never have met if it weren't for this book.

They are my muses.

HUGE thanks to Christina Lianos (page 77), whose tireless efforts helped make this book a reality.

Special thanks to David Storey, who persuaded me to try paleo, and to Jamil Moledina (page 95) and Brent Britton, my consiglieres throughout this project.

Thanks also to Karen Pendergrass (a.k.a. "The Paleo Queen", page 146) and Tim Swart (a.k.a "Dr. Bacon", page 165) and all the rest of the brilliant, warm, positive, and supporting members, physicians, scientists, nutritionists, fitness gurus, dietitians, and bodybuilders in IPMG, The International Paleo Movement Group, on Facebook (http://is.gd/paleogroup), far too numerous to list here, whose collective advice helped me change my life.

Thanks to Edward Cantrell for maintaining the information and links at http://is.gd/paleo

Finally, thanks to everyone featured in this book for their courage, inspiration, and common desire to help save lives and change the world for the better.

IT'S *YOUR* CHOICE

Paleo is more than just a way of eating. It is a philosophy with the following premise:

Take nothing for granted, do your own research about nutrition, eat clean natural unprocessed foods, and listen to your body.

If you dig deeply enough into the studies that have been done about nutrition, you will come across a lot of information that contravenes contemporary "wisdom" about fat, carbs, and protein, and which sources of these are best for your body. You will learn about lectins, anti-nutrients, and bioavailability.

Unlike other "diets," the paleo list of foods to stay away from is not a random selection the author of the diet believes will prevent you from getting fat. We in the Paleo community do not eat certain foods because we believe, based on both our research and our experiences, that they are poisonous to our bodies.

So what are these foods? Grains, processed foods, sugars, vegetable oils, beans, potatoes, and for some of us, dairy. It's a short list - but these foods make up an increasingly larger percentage of the Standard American Diet ("SAD"), and consumption of them is at an all-time historical high. At the same time, the rates of heart disease, high blood pressure, cancer, diabetes, celiac disease, anxiety disorders, and countless others, are also at an all-time high.

But, if you do a good job researching, you will learn that correlation does not equal causation. And that is why I put this book together: To connect the dots for you.

Many of those who eat paleo do so simply because it makes them feel younger, more lucid, more energetic, and they love how they look naked.

On the other hand, many of us have been forced to do so because we had a disease or condition. We were dissatisfied with what we were told by our physicians was the only option: Living with an incurable disease because it is genetic, and managing the symptoms with expensive prescription medicine.

In the paleo community, we believe that FOOD IS MEDICINE. We have either eliminated all symptoms of, or dramatically improved, the diseases we had by eating REAL food - as much of it as our hearts desire - and in most cases have become completely medication-free. And we have also learned that when your body is healthy inside, it looks healthier on the outside too. As a result, most of us have dropped weight or have experienced a shift of weight away from the less flattering parts of our bodies. Bonus.

The people featured in this book have all undergone an inspiring transformation, to the point where many of them have started blogs or websites, and written books. We are all born again, and are excited to share our secret with you.

After reading the stories contained in this book, you will make a choice.

On the one hand, you can read this book, mentally categorize it as too good to be true, and continue eating a SAD diet because you like how good it tastes, or because that is what you were told to do. Most of you will select this choice because, quite frankly, it easier to continue believing what you already believe - besides, you really like your cereal, pasta, and whole grain bread. You will no longer wonder why, despite that you are eating what most people consider to be healthy, and are doing tons of cardio, your health and fitness have plateaued or declined. You will just chalk it up to age or genetics.

On the other hand, if you have the courage to put yourself to the task, and are willing to get through 2-3 tough weeks of tough transition and grain withdrawal while you infuse your body with healthy fats, clean carbs, and lots of nutrients, you may discover what has been described as the fountain of youth, dramatically improve medical conditions that you have been managing your whole life, and drop weight as you never thought possible.

And although we in the paleo community have all done it, it is nonetheless nothing short of a true miracle.

So there it is. Choose wisely...because you are the one who has to live with the results of your choice for the rest of your life.

Peace and love to all,

Joseph Salama
November 3, 2012

STORIES:

THE PALEO MIRACLE

BILL VICK

PLANO, TEXAS

www.ifitboomer.com

Growing up, like most of us, I was always involved in sports. In high school it was wrestling, and later on running, swimming, karate and the martial arts. I joined the Marine Corps and was accepted into Force Recon, an elite group that is focused on long-range reconnaissance.

After I got married and had children, I stopped paying attention to my health and all but stopped any regular exercise. To get back in shape, I started working out including some masters swimming and running. I never smoked, I never did drugs, and I thought I did everything "right" from a diet perspective. Or so I thought. My diet was a grain-based high carbohydrate diet, the Standard American Diet (SAD) diet.

A year ago, as I was swimming in training for short course triathlon, I found that I was out of breath and I had a persistent cough that didn't seem to want to go away. My first thought was that I had developed asthma or COPD. So I decided to go see my doctor.

In September 2011, my primary physician ran some tests, and then referred me to a pulmonologist who diagnosed me with Idiopathic Pulmonary Fibrosis (IPF). I was told that IPF is a disease where the lungs scar and stiffen, and that it primarily attacks people 50 years old and over. I was told that when that lung tissue dies, it doesn't grow back, it is gone for good. I was told that the best hope for people with IPF is commonly thought to be a lung transplant and there is no treatment on the near or far horizon.

Like most people, I had never heard of IPF so I started researching it and learned there are over 200,000 people in the US who have it, 48,000 people are diagnosed each year and 40,000 people die from it annually, or one every 13 minutes. The life expectancy after diagnosis is typically three to five years. There is no known cure. If you get it you die. It's just a matter of when. The general consensus is that it is primarily an autoimmune response, a disease caused by the body's own defense mechanisms in response to some stimuli. IPF is typically treated with heavy-duty immune system suppressing drugs like prednisone, but the drugs don't address the underlying cause, they only help manage the symptoms. Funding for research is negligible.

I was training as a triathlete, I looked good, I felt good, and my life was on track. I couldn't believe that this was happening to me at first and was not given any hope by my doctors. I continued to do research on my own – eventually reading Mark Sisson's *The Primal Blueprint*, Robb Wolf's *The Paleo Solution*, and Loren Cordain's *The Paleo Diet*. The more I read, the more convinced I became that an autoimmune disease could be treated effectively through proper diet and lifestyle. I learned that the paleo diet specifically addresses the autoimmune responses of the body. It made sense to me, but I wasn't ready to start yet. I went to see one of the leading pulmonologists in the world at National Jewish Health in Denver to discuss diet with him. I told him about everything I had learned about paleo and why it made sense that it should work – and much to my surprise, he thought it was worth a try and encouraged me to try it since nothing else was really available.

Shortly after I made the switch to the paleo lifestyle, my IPF stabilized (which is as good as it gets). It has now been under control for over six months. I was previously on medication for high cholesterol (statins), acid reflux, and depression. After a mere two months of paleo I was able to stop all of the medications.

I have since come to accept my situation. My IPF is not cured – I am still living with it but now I can live my life fully, and do not have to be a victim of it. Paleo has literally saved my life.

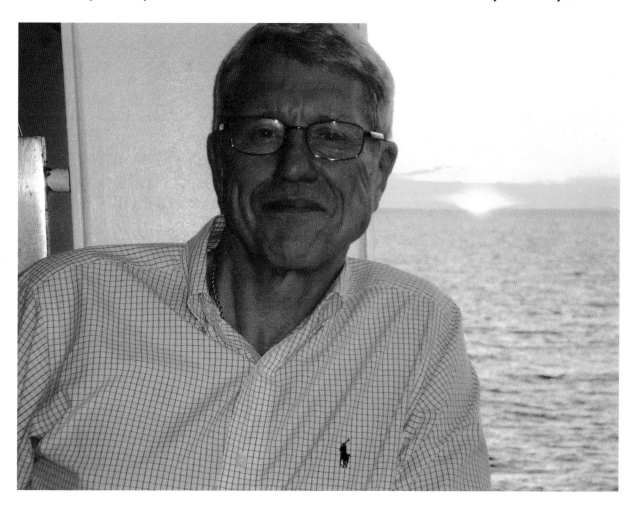

I still have some anger inside me though. I'm angry that IPF has no known cure. I am angry that most Americans are ignorant about IPF – which kills as many people as lung cancer does every year, but gets no attention. That is why my goal now is to help spread awareness of IPF – which is one of the reasons I wanted to be in this book. There will not be enough money going into the necessary research needed to find a cure until there is more public awareness. If I educate just one more person about IPF, and if one person who has IPF can learn from my story, then I have accomplished my goal.

To that end, I have put up several websites including BoomerJobTips.com focused on boomer careers, and iFitBoomer.com focused on boomer fitness to help boomers in their lives. I firmly believe that the cultivation of crops like wheat, barley, corn, legumes, rice, and potatoes not only altered our diets, but brought with it the so-called diseases of affluence, and I want to help as many people understand living well is possible regardless of your age or having a disease like IPF.

I am now 74 years old and no longer run triathlons competitively but I am training for and entering masters swimming and running events. I no longer compete with others but I do compete with myself daily and strive to be the best I can be. But if you see me out there in the pool or on the track, be sure to say hello and remember to live each day because that is the only day you have.

LISA ENDRES

BERKELEY HEIGHTS, NEW JERSEY

My journey towards finding the paleo lifestyle started 6 years ago in 2006. I was 39 years old, 195 pounds, with over 50% body fat. I was having severe pounding headaches, had some difficulty breathing on exertion, was tired all the time, and experiencing gastric reflux at night. I chalked it up to more of a psychological etiology – and to having 3 children. I was feeling horrible all the time. I had been depending mostly on frozen entrees, fast food, and meals that could be quickly thrown together to feed myself and my family. A typical breakfast was bagels/breads, muffins, cereal, sugary oatmeal, or frozen waffles. Lunch consisted of sandwiches made with deli meats and cheeses or the old standby of peanut butter and jelly. Snacks were chips, cookies, or goldfish crackers, maybe a piece of fruit. We would go days without a vegetable - maybe a salad if it came with the entrée at a restaurant. And dinner would be pasta or a family sized frozen tray of something ready to just put in the oven. Dessert – there was always dessert – typically a cake or ice cream.

I was also feeding myself negative thoughts of not being a good enough mother and not being able to "handle it" like everyone else around me. Over time my symptoms worsened, and I began getting dizzy when walking up a flight of stairs. Finally, one day, I ultimately passed out. After this happened a few times, and I began to experience a slight on and off pinching sensation in the area of my heart, I realized something was wrong, and went to a cardiologist.

Upon initial examination, he discovered that my heart rate was over 100 beats per minute, my blood pressure was 188/118 and I was pale in color. He also did an EKG, and immediately put me on several medications: Captopril, Diovan HCT, and Toprol XL. He was very straightforward and told me that he could already tell, without the results of tests he was planning on scheduling, that I was very sick and if I wanted to see my three little girls grow up, that I needed to make a change immediately. He suggested a few popular weight loss programs. I was scared straight into joining one the very next day. He also scheduled other tests – a stress test and an echocardiogram with contrast. I remember the day of the stress test very vividly. I was only able to walk on the treadmill for 90 seconds at 2.0 mph with a slight incline before feeling dizzy and having to be escorted to the examination table nearby to lay down. He informed me that I should not start any exercise regime yet, and to only concentrate on changing my nutritional habits until he was able to further diagnose me.

When I first started my weight loss program, I incorporated fruits and vegetables into my day. I bought no-fat everything and a lot of whole grain-rich foods. But I continued to buy frozen meals, just ones that were more portion-controlled and calorie-friendly.

After a couple of weeks, I received word that I had three severely leaky valves and the walls of the four heart chambers were thickened. What this meant was that the chambers themselves were receiving a lesser volume of blood, and what it was receiving was back flowing because the valves were faulty. The blood, in turn, backed up to my lungs, which was causing me to be short of breath. There was not an efficient circulation of blood, so I was being deprived of oxygen to my brain (dizziness) and to my tissues (pale color). My cardiologist informed me that I did suffer some permanent damage to my heart. And then he said it – Congestive Heart Failure. He started talking about surgery as an option. It was not his first choice, but he was going to monitor me very closely and give my weight loss program a chance to work. I really thought I was going to die.

I was able to start exercising after 3 months of "dieting" in late winter of 2007. I mostly walked on the treadmill and then advanced to group classes, some with light weights, at a gym. I also used the machines in the weight room and the pool, albeit infrequently. I did some form of mild exercise everyday between 30 and 60 minutes. It took me one year and seven months to lose 70 pounds, and finally attained my goal weight in June 2008. I was then 125 pounds, but I was still 30% fat and had dimpled skin, looked saggy, and my face was somewhat drawn. I was happy how my body looked in clothes, but not out of them. I certainly looked better than how I did before, so I chose to concentrate on the positive and accept that I was now in my 40s and had 3 pregnancies and my rippled tummy was a fact of life. Many of my physical symptoms had dissipated, but the disheartening part was that my blood lab values had not changed much. My cholesterol still lingered around 180mg/dL, and triglycerides and LDL's were still elevated. I was also feeling weak, cranky and hungry all the time.

After maintaining this until September of 2009, the weight started creeping back on, until I was up to 140 pounds. In January 2010, I started at another gym, by a friend's recommendation, and was introduced to lifting heavy with free weights, kettle bells, pulling sleds, pushing prowlers, HIIT and density training. Nutrition was a major part of their program – and this is where I first heard about the paleo diet. I had an amazing trainer, who was knowledgeable, motivating, and passionate about his job and teaching others. He recommended I try paleo during an 8-week fat-loss competition the gym was running. I trusted him implicitly and I gave it a try.

The competition ran from March to May of 2010. Improvement was noticeable to me in 4 weeks. But after 8 weeks, my rippled tummy was gone! My fat percentage went from 27.2% to 23.5% and I lost 5 pounds of pure fat while maintaining all of my muscle mass. So I was back down to 125 pounds, but only 23.5% fat instead of the 30% on that previous weight loss program. I began to understand that losing weight is not the same thing as losing fat, and eating more protein and moderate healthy fats gave me much more energy, concentration, and just an all around vibrant feeling.

A few months later, I went to have more blood work done, and was excited to tell my doctor of my new lifestyle. He cringed when he heard how many eggs and portions of red meat I was eating. But when my results came back he said, "I can't tell you to stop what you are doing, because whatever it is, it's working." My cholesterol had dropped to 126mg/dl, my blood pressure was 110/68mmHg, my triglycerides and LDLs were way down, and HDLs were elevated. All great news! Cutting out grains, dairy, legumes, and all processed foods also allowed me to get off 3 of the 4 medications that I was taking! It wasn't the large weight loss

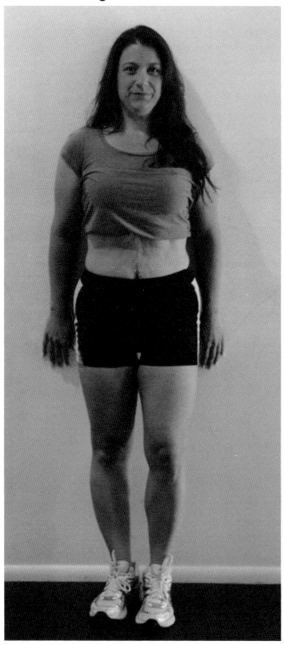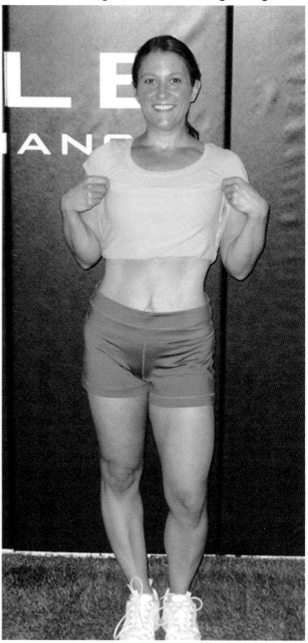

(photo courtesy Gabriele Fitness & Performance, www.gabrielefitness.com) that really helped me, it was the FOODS I was choosing to put in my body.

I have continued the paleo lifestyle for 2 ½ years now. I converted my whole family over about 9 months ago. I'm not going to lie: it was hard. But knowing it is the best thing for every one, I dug my heels in and didn't give in to the whining, moaning and complaining. It gets worse before it gets better, but at some point they reach their saturation level and realize things are not going to change. You just have to hold your ground. My three daughters, ages 15, 11, and 9 now love to come with me to the farmer's market to pick out the vegetables they like. They also enjoy helping me prepare meals, going through my paleo cookbooks or even researching recipes on the internet for us to try. It is also a great bonding experience for us, and we are openly able to discuss being healthy and having strong bodies. They have also begun to recognize the benefits of their eating, such as increased athletic performance, concentration, strength and endurance during activities, and improved alertness and mood.

I am still attending the same gym, do weight training 2 – 3 times per week. At 45 years old, I am 131 pounds and down to 17.6% body fat, and falling. The 6 pound gain does not bother me because I feel and look better in my clothes, and I am leaner and more defined and feel more vibrant than I have in decades. I feel passionate about life again, which has also overflowed and improved all the relationships in my life. For me, it has been a whole mind, body, soul reconnection – and it feels absolutely wonderful!

TERESA

COOL, CALIFORNIA

My first desire in all of this was to lose weight. At the age of 31, I was 5', 2" and 125 pounds. A decent weight, but "skinny fat," despite being active and having a regular exercise routine. By age 46 I weighed 210 pounds. During the last twelve years, I attempted to change my eating patterns with the help of health and nutrition professionals and other popular weight loss programs, but all methods failed to achieve any significant or long term results.

At the age of 31, at 5', 2" 125 pounds, I temporarily became a closet binge eater during my engagement and wedding planning year, and thus began my never ending battle with weight gain. Don't we all wish to look the ideal part of the gorgeous blushing bride? In my first three months of wedding planning I managed to gain 15 pounds before I sought professional help. I visited a medical doctor specializing in weight loss. In order to restore my girly figure, the first thing we tried were Phentermine pills. Next was an expensive line of pre-packaged, high protein, additive-loaded food products sold only by the physician's office. The smallish-boxed items weren't exactly foods, but were mostly tasteless, powdered soups and other powdered fake foods, to simulate a popular high-protein, low-carb diet. By day three of my medically approved diet, I realized I was experiencing nasty, rare side effects from Phentermine. So I returned to the doctor's office. The doctor advised I stop taking Phentermine, but not without expressing how disappointed he was that I would no longer be able to take it. The physician's disappointment, I suspect, stemmed from the fact that the real success of his business was selling Phentermine – being that Phentermine greatly reduces appetite and most people who take it just stop eating completely. My next (and final) failure came from not being able to choke down that awful powdered boxed food, and the approved daily salad was not enough to curb my hunger pangs without the Phentermine. I was starving and the powdered food plan left me wanting to sneak other food and I did eat off plan. I was cranky, irritable, low in energy, miserable, and everyone around me was victim to my irritability.

During my medically supervised diet, I had been exercising three to four hours a day, five days a week. My daily minimal exercise routine consisted of one hour of cardio, one hour of weight lifting, one hour of tennis, and on some days one hour of walking. I was determined to lose my 15 pounds and another 10 pounds before my wedding day. According to the doctor, my loss of 1.5 pound per week was too slow. After my second month of weekly office visits, the doctor suggested I again try Phentermine. That day I left his office, never to return. I realized a medically supervised diet is not necessarily safe or healthy. I maintained my exercise routine until my wedding day, and I managed to lose the 15 pounds from limiting my closet binge eating. I lost inches from my continued exercise, allowing me to fit into a smaller size 10 gown (instead of size 12), but I was still "skinny fat" and still unhappy with my appearance. I also knew my work out routine would not be a lifelong plan.

I settled into marriage, decreased my exercise to three times a week for 1-1.5 hours a day, and slowly started to gain weight over the next 4 years. At 36 years of age, and at my all-time highest weight of 145 pounds, more than my last day of full term pregnancy, I sought the help of a naturopathic doctor. The goal was now to take a truck-load of expensive vitamins before, during and after each meal. After the second month, the cases of vitamins were cost-prohibitive and I stopped altogether. That was the end of that plan.

Between ages of 36 and 40 I also started a diet where I counted points for a few short months. I couldn't reliably keep track of how many points a single serving of my homemade dishes were. I also could not monitor points for dishes that had no attached point system. The pre-packed frozen meals were always so skimpy and filled with a ton of additives. This method lasted two months with no resulting weight loss. It was all so complicated and sometimes I just wanted to eat and not overanalyze the point system or calorie of each bite. Also, with all these plans, I never felt satiated, energetic, or excited about my food options, and I never really had significant weight loss without some intense exercise routine. At one point I decided I wasn't failing, but that my genetic make-up was failing me and I was destined to forever be fat. That was my excuse and I stuck by it for six more years. I stopped my regular exercise routine at age 42.

When I turned 43 years old I weighed 200 pounds. Never did I ever believe I would tip the scales at 150 pounds, let alone 200. And that wasn't even the worst of all of my weight gain or health issues. I was feeling depressed long before I reached 200 pounds. I stopped attending social functions out of embarrassment with my appearance and fear of criticism from others about my rapid weight gain. I refused to have my picture taken. I couldn't move with the same speed or agility from when I weighed less. I loathed shopping for clothes. The nearby mall had approximately 70 women's fashion stores, but only 4 stores where I could find women's clothing in my size. I also suffered from GERD, Irritable Bowel Syndrome, the start of an irregular menstrual cycle with increasing PMS symptoms, and severe upper back and neck inflammation which caused headaches and pain which prevented me from sleeping.

I also participated in the free employer sponsored bio-metric health screening to lower my health insurance costs. I didn't expect the results I got. I had always been in the healthy range, but now my lipid panel showed that I was high risk for a stroke, heart attack, was pre-diabetic with metabolic syndrome, and the list kept going. My mother, at age 50, suffered multiple strokes within a two-month time span, had a stent placed, and I knew my near future years were leading me down the same stroke path if I did not make a change before I turned 50. So I scheduled an appointment with my family doctor.

My doctor was more than willing to help suggest ways to lose weight and reduce my stroke risk. Unfortunately, the doctor's first recommendation was Phentermine. No way! The doctor's second recommendation was to seek counseling from a nutritionist. With high hopes, I began to meet once a week for almost seven months with a nutritionist. The plan was to follow the USDA food pyramid to the letter and to return to a regular cardio exercise routine. The plan seemed to start well. In the first month I lost 5 pounds. In the second month I lost 2 pounds. Then, over the next five months I couldn't shed a single pound no matter how committed I was and no matter how much I exercised. I was stuck indefinitely at 193 pounds and I felt as if I was at a dead end. The final straw came near the end of my six months when the nutritionist chastised me for my avocado snack. "Do you realize how much fat is in an avocado and how unhealthy avocados are compared to bread? You should have eaten bread." There is something inherently misplaced about valuing foods with unrecognizable chemical additives (like bread) as more healthy than whole natural foods (like avocados). My health did not improve and my lipid panels did not show any reversal of change. In fact, my lipid panels got worse. The doctor wanted to prescribe statins. I refused the statins, believing I could eat my way to health, but I didn't know how or what to eat to make this happen.

But still, even following the nutritionist's consultation, I remained high risk for stroke, heart attack, and pre-diabetic. I still had metabolic syndrome. My daily blood sugar changes were like a roller coaster. I was crashing all day long. My IBS and GERD worsened, and my menstrual cycle was really whacked – and my doctor insisted that my irregular menstrual cycle change was related to age, not health. I believed that it was genetics that made me fat and lethargic. Worse, I lost all hope that I could ever be healthy again. If professionals couldn't help, then there was no hope for me. So, I gave up. I ate a pint of ice cream in a single sitting more than once a week. I let my health deteriorate over the next three years and I remained depressed because of my weight and health. Occasionally I entertained gastric-bypass type surgery, but I feared any long term, permanent consequences.

Fast forward to age 46. I now tipped the scale at a new all-time high of 210 pounds as of November 2011. In December, my son invited me to his high school Mother-Son, Father-Daughter dance to be held the following month. The theme was the Roaring 20s. I shopped and shopped for a dress in my size, but I could not fit into a 3X sized dress. I had not even worn a dress in eight years. By then I had started to research paleo, and for several months I read online testimonials of how ancestral eating helped others not only lose weight, but how others relieved their IBS, GERD, lowered their lipid panels, etc., simply by eating the right foods. To be honest, I was skeptical of all these health change claims.

One morning I received a horrible phone call. My mother's youngest brother, my uncle, then 55, had suffered a series of strokes and was hospitalized. Similar to my mother's experience, he too had a stent placed. My uncle's unfortunate health crisis encouraged me to explore paleo, and I began my journey on January 17, 2012.

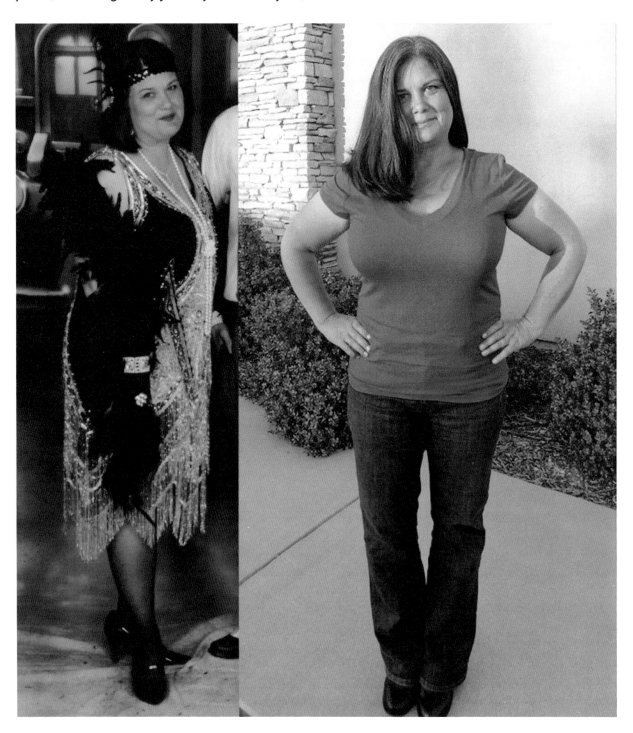

I recently turned 47, and instead of reaching another all-time weight gain record, I trimmed down 36 pounds without exercise, while eating tons of food. I can't even believe how much food I eat. A typical day consists of five eggs for breakfast, sometimes two pieces of bacon. For lunch, I either have a large salad with tuna or a beef patty. Dinner tends to be a 10 oz steak or wild caught fish with one or two sides of vegetables. My current weight is 174 pounds and I am rocking a new me for the first time in almost a decade. A few months before I couldn't fit into a size 3X dress, I wore a size 20W in pants, a 3X in tops…and now I wear a size 14 regular in pants and L and XL in tops. I lost 8 inches from my abdomen, another 8 inches from my hips, and 7 inches from my chest measurements. And that's not even the best part of my journey.

Within the first weeks of changing to ancestral eating my daily GERD and IBS disappeared. My menstrual cycle is no longer irregular, and has returned to pre-pregnancy normalness. My lifelong affliction with PMS has improved, a very unexpected and desirable change, and I no longer have symptoms of irritability and lethargy 2 weeks before I start my cycle. I used to measure my cycle by my symptoms, and now I need to use a calendar. For the past three years I have suffered extreme upper back and neck inflammation, which then caused a nasty headache and impaired me from regular activities whether work or home related. In the past 2 years, the inflammatory pain caused me to have difficulty sleeping. Medication would dull the pain, but not eliminate the pain and my headaches persisted. The medication only mitigated some of the symptoms. But with paleo eating the inflammation has been cured, and only returns if I eat grains or food additives. I never realized how much the daily pain was changing my outlook on life. I am no longer on a sugar high and crash program. I have so much more energy and clarity of mind than my past years I am amazed at how great I feel.

The most exciting part of my journey is my lipid profile. Just shy of 2 months of being paleo, I participated in my employer sponsored bio-metric screening, because I wanted to put the "high saturated fat is bad for you" issue to bed forever. When my numbers came in, I was elated by what they revealed. I was no longer pre-diabetic, I no longer had metabolic syndrome. My 2009 triglycerides were 234 mg/dl. After a mere 2 months of ancestral eating my triglycerides dropped to 134 mg/dl. My 2009 HDL was 38 mg/dl, in the unhealthy-low range, and my 2012 HDL was 50 mg/dl. I was certainly surprised by the improved changes. I had little weight difference. The bad LDL particle size changed from a small dense size of 6.15 to a larger, buoyant particle size of 2.68, approximating the 2.0 healthy range. In 2009 the nurse recorded my weight at 196 pounds. In 2012 my recorded weight was 191 pounds.

I am still on my weight loss journey, but I am also now developing my own personal paleo template to fit my body type in order to continually improve my overall health. I won't lie – my biggest hurdle was overcoming my addiction to grains. I learned my addiction was not carb-based, but sugar-based. During my third month of ancestral eating I cut all sugars for 30 days to overcome my sugar addiction. As a result, I stopped craving processed bread type foods. Kicking my daily need for sugar has been difficult, but very rewarding.

Improving my health has become my number one priority, more so now that I know I can master my desired changes without drugs, but with pure, whole foods. I still have my pint of ice cream once or twice a month. Although now I eat an organic, additive free ice cream about twice a month, or make a delicious homemade coconut milk ice cream. I no longer fear being seen by others, and I am beginning a new exercise routine through my employer. In the next few months I will again have another bio-metric screening and I am very excited to see my next results.

AARON RENTFREW

MIAMI BEACH, FLORIDA

www.sobeprimal.com

I have always been the type to pick something up, use it vigorously, and then put it back on the shelf in favor of the next best thing. For most of my life, my attempts at achieving a healthy lifestyle were no exception. Over time, I've been through a wide range of physical conditions. Like many good Jersey boys, in high school I found myself in a crowd of jocks, always in the gym and eating tons of carbs and protein. As time went on, staying in shape turned into an afterthought as everyday concerns like paying bills, working, and the exciting world of parties and booze took over all my available time.

I was of the lucky variety that can hold onto a leaner physique, even with minimal working out and an awful diet. This "luck" kept me out of the gym sometimes for years at a time, letting my musculature wither away until guilt and shame would slowly give me the spark to start doing pushups, which I would immediately gloat about to my friends: "I started working out again today, I feel MUCH better," I would say, awarding myself a nice big pat on the back and a spaghetti dinner to celebrate my newfound workout ethic. Within a week, a month, whatever, I'd be back to my old routine of work, drink, sleep, repeat. There were many squandered gym memberships and countless broken promises that somehow I was going to dramatically reinvent myself. I would switch my diet up to "healthy" stuff like cereal, whole grains, and other complex carbs, which was easy because I literally could not get enough of them, and take to cooking with canola oil or consuming basically no fat at all.

Over the last few years things began to weigh heavily on me. A mixture of fatigue, stress, and an overall lack of wellness mentally and physically made it harder to get through the day. I felt as though I was REALLY ready for some sort of change. The first thing that I chose to cut out was alcohol (might be drastic for some, but for me it was a necessity), and then I began working out at a gym — still without making much of a change in my diet.

I got my strength back relatively quickly and actually began to put on some size (still with a lingering "spare tire" around my midsection). This went on for about four months until the gains stopped. Fat was no longer exiting my body, and my workouts began to stagnate. Once the gains stopped, I wanted to stop.

Luckily, a friend came into my life at just the right time. He was a crossfitting, softball-playing, power-lifting ball of energy. He began to preach about the dangers of grains and pushed me into trying other forms of workouts. I must admit I was very skeptical about the "dangers" of cereal and whole grains, even though his explanations did seem to make perfect sense. After all, this really flew in the face of my previous understanding of a well balanced diet, consisting of nine to 11 servings a day of grains, coupled with minimal fat. I thought for sure that I was simply not working out hard enough, or that maybe I should eat less. I was sure this high-fat, no-grain diet would make me break out with pimples, get fat, and lose muscle mass. Looking back, I'm not sure why I was afraid of these things…but I was.

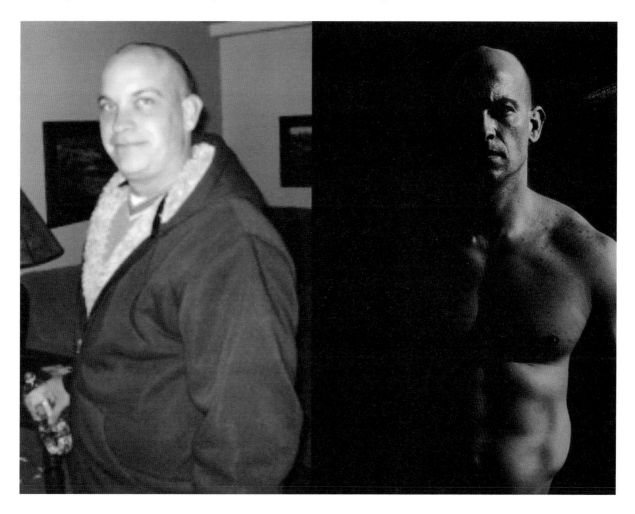

Finally… I was fed up with my stunted muscle growth, and that, combined with the fact that I couldn't lose my fatty midsection, brought me to a turning point: I was willing to try the "paleo diet." After about a week or two, all cravings for things sweet, starchy, cereal-y, and grainy were all gone. I found a variety of fruits and veggies that I never knew I liked, and have now come to love. I have begun rendering my own animal fat for cooking instead of the assortment of oils readily available at the local market.

And the "diet" is just the beginning. I have created my own workouts, which I do outside in the sun, and they are a thousand times better than anything the gym has to offer. Nearly every day I am out enjoying our beautiful tropical climate in Miami Beach, whereas before I was most often holing up in some gray climate-controlled room. What I will say now, though, is that the excess fat is gone, my mood is better than ever, my skin is tanned, and I feel as though I have found a style of living that I will enjoy for years to come.

I have found myself in the best relationship ever with a woman that loves to eat a paleo diet. We cook together, eat together, and workout together. Health is quite contagious. She is a "recovering" ballet dancer who has been on extreme diets her entire life and had a host of health issues because of it. She was downright terrified of fat when I told her the food I eat. But, as with most people I come in contact with, she eventually got past her prior prejudice because I have proven by example that this whole "eat real food" thing works magic.

Not to be cliché, but it's the simple truth: I have NEVER felt better. I hope that others will come to reap the benefits this paleo way of life as well. It has been a godsend for me, and many others I have come to know. Everywhere I go, my friends ask me about what I am doing to stay fit. As more and more of them begin incorporating elements of the paleo lifestyle into their own, I witness in them the positive changes I have experienced myself, and it drives me to spread the word further as I continue to carve out my own paleo path.

CRISTA

MIAMI, FLORIDA

Both of my parents came from poor families before they turned themselves into legends in their fields despite the odds and hardships that they faced on the way. To scratch the surface of their achievements in life, my mother was an Olympic figure skater and my father was the most famous American male ballet dancer who ever lived.

I grew up watching my parents being given medals by presidents and meeting famous people at galas. I was always asked if I was going to be a dancer like my dad one day. "Yes," I would say. I wanted to be a dancer. I thought it was my birthright to pass on the legacy of my father. It seemed as if those were the expectations that were placed on me, and I certainly placed those expectations on myself. I was born with a talent to match my parents, a drive to live up to my family name, and a belief that if my parents could do it coming from their backgrounds that I had no excuse to be anything less than they were. The bar was set so impossibly high that every accomplishment in my life seemed distant by comparison.

Despite what I inherited, there were other variables that got in the way of my lofty goals. One big one in particular was my body. I only reached 5', 1" tall and I had a naturally muscular physique. I never developed into the long, elegant, naturally thin woman that is required of the level of ballerina that I wanted to be.

So I dieted. Fat became my worst enemy. Fat was the evil keeping me from living my dreams. I studied food labels and didn't touch anything with a mere gram of fat in it. I stopped eating fat at the age 14. I even got thin, but not from a lack of fat grams, but because I starved myself. My fat depletion caused me health problems because fat has many valuable functions in the human body that I didn't know about then. In my extreme "no fat years" as a teenager, I weighed from 70 to 85 pounds. I stopped getting my period. I had severe problems with constipation that left me so toxic that doctors feared for my life. I was cold all of the time. I was irritable. I had no energy. And I had few friends.

I eventually pulled my head together and became what I thought of as a very healthy person mentally, physically and spiritually. I stopped dancing and went to NYU. I continued exercising regularly and I ate what the mainstream would consider to be a very "healthy low fat diet." I weighed between 101 to 105 pounds, and was frequently complimented on my great body.

There was only one health problem left. I still never got regular periods. I would go on average 3 to 4 months in between periods. Doctors informed me that this was normal for active women and I didn't complain or worry because on some level it seemed like a perk.

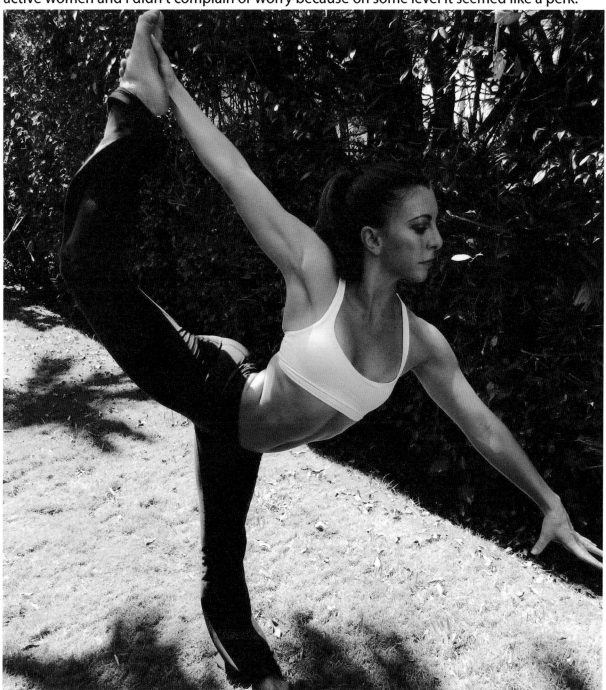

The next "health issue" came in my late 20s. I went to my therapist to help me cope with the stress of an amazing but overwhelming job that I didn't want to give up. I was diagnosed with ADHD and I reluctantly took the prescribed meds – prescription amphetamines - because it seemed to really help me on the job.

A few years later, I met my current boyfriend Aaron Rentfrew. He is the guy I have been always searching for my whole life, and he is totally paleo! He has a calm demeanor, a great body, and an incredible outlook on life. He glows and he makes me very happy. He started selling me on paleo right away. But I still had some deep, hidden fears from my past about eating a high fat diet.

I couldn't believe in it, despite his ample evidence and the living proof he was of its success. I thought that it may work for guys, but that there was no way that a girl could eat that much fat and still look great. I had worked so hard to get my body and my body image in order. I liked myself and I didn't want to tip the boat. But alas, he is a great cook!!! And he would make me all of these amazing Paleo meals! And, I was in love! And every time I expressed a fat concern, he would disprove me with Paleo facts! If I wasn't so in love, I would have never listened, but I told myself, "When I gain 5 pounds, I will stop eating this high fat diet and lose the weight again." Until then, I was going to try and trust him because it was so much fun to eat with him.

Well, the chance I took really paid off. I have been paleo for over a year now, and I never gained a pound. I weigh exactly what I weighed in college, but I eat more, I am healthier, and I worry less! I get my period regularly now. My skin glows and my hair is shinier. I am happier and more energetic. I have gotten off of all of my ADHD medication and my concentration no longer seems to be a problem. I am doing great at work. I needed more fat in my diet.

Paleo has given me the physical, spiritual, and mental health that I have always searched for and struggled so hard to achieve. I am so grateful to be able to relax, eat, love my body, and feel healthier than ever. Being paleo has enabled me to really be who I want to be... a healthy woman with a great body, self-love, and serenity. My relationship with food is so much easier and healthier now than ever before. I hope that all women in unhealthy relationships with food can find the courage to change their lives by being true to their nature and finding a healthy paleo relationship. It won't make you fat. I promise.

NICK BENCIVENGA

SAN FRANCISCO, CALIFORNIA

benci007@gmail.com

I always considered myself to be at least *conscious* of my health. I was never "fat," but I never felt in-shape either. My single mother was very health conscious, and that included being vegetarian. Although I ate meat, it was sparse and not a staple. I ate a lot of baguette and pasta. When I was in my teen years, I moved in with my father. This included a steady intake of junk food: Frozen foods, crackers, chips, soda, juice, cereal, candy, etc. It added up. When I left for college, I was 6'2", 180 pounds. I felt decent, but I always had a little "spare tire" around my belly.

As I went through college, things only went downhill. My first two years consisted of a lot of beer and fast food. Taco Bell, McDonalds, pizza, and frozen meals were the regular meals in our apartment. I was pretty abusive to my body with respect to alcohol in particular. When I reflect on this time, although there was a lot of laughter, there is embarrassment and shame. But, it is what it is, and I gained weight regularly. I was usually hovering around 190-195 pounds. I carried it well, and never looked "fat" – but I never felt confident in my looks. I hated having to take my shirt off. I always felt like I had to "suck in" and was constantly envious of any guy with a six-pack. It was frustrating. I never felt good. My sleep patterns were terrible. I'd have indigestion, nausea in the mornings, and constant unease. I wrote everything off as "drinking too much" which was probably true in part – but in retrospect, food was definitely a culprit.

When I left college at age 21, I was around 190 pounds, and headed to California. I went with my best friend, who is gifted with a fast metabolism and a penchant for sports. He's about 5'7", and 140 pounds, very muscular and athletic. He never has to try to be skinny. We spent almost a month on a road trip across the country, and when we got to California, I felt like garbage when I looked at the photos of both of us with our shirts off. I felt weak and fat, as usual. My life in California continued my bad habits – beer, food excess, and a general lack of care for my general well-being.

A few years after meeting my eventual wife, we decided to move to Korea for a year to teach English together. It was one of the best years of my life. While in Seoul, I started unintentionally becoming Paleo. Koreans love fermented foods, fresh meat, and they limit grains and gluten. The only "bad" thing in the diet is white rice, which by most Paleo standards is one of the "less bad" grains. So while we were there, we started eating a little better. My alcohol intake went down. And finally, we decided that we wanted to exercise more seriously. We went through the "Insanity" program, and although a bit intense, we felt the results, and I started to lose a little bit of weight. I was feeling muscular, and liking how I looked. My interest in health was piqued, so I started reading a bit. I read some Michael Pollan, and things started clicking a little bit. I wasn't Paleo, but I was using my brain. A good start.

We came back to San Francisco and I was feeling decent, but not great. I still had indigestion.

I still didn't sleep well. As we re-connected with friends, we started falling back into old habits. I still couldn't get rid of that tire around my belly. Then, I got lucky. My moment. A friend messaged me on Facebook about Mark's Daily Apple. I clicked that link… and my life has never been the same since. I poured through every article, story, testament, and link he had to offer. It was amazing. Everything started to make sense. I was hooked. My wife… not so

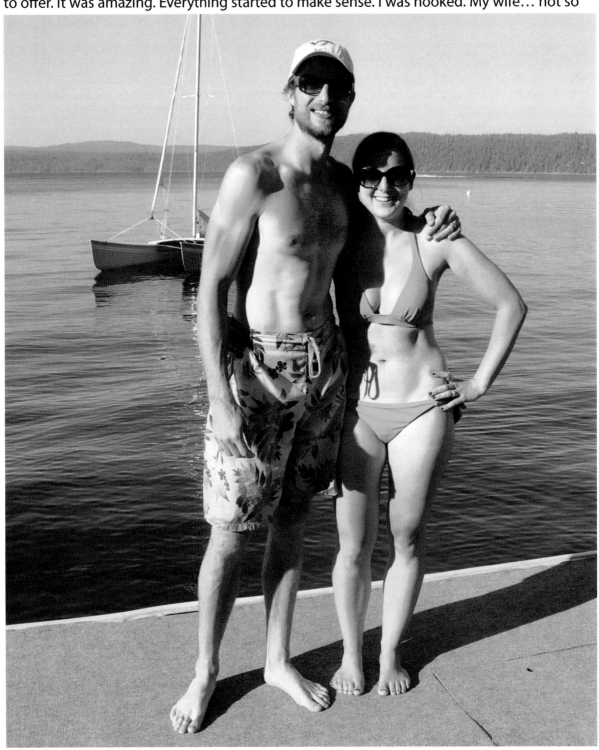

much. It took about a week of my yammering to get her to sign on to switch her cooking. We decided to do 30 days together, cutting out all grains and sugar. The results were incredible.

I felt so light. So energetic. So… right. Don't get me wrong, the first week was tough. I wanted sugar, and I wanted it bad. But that passed, and quick. We started eating bacon. We started eating lots of butter. Lots of fish, beef, chicken. Meat in general. We stopped feeling guilty when we saw the word "fat" on the package. We stopped buying things in packages. The change was almost immediate. Within the first few days the top layer of fat on my body almost melted away. I was losing a few pounds a week. I eventually settled out around 155-160 pounds, on my 6'2" frame. I'm pretty muscular, and have stayed at this weight for well over a year now.

It's been about a year and a half now since I've made the switch, and I don't think I'll ever go back. Every time I break the rules, I feel like garbage. So, I stick pretty close to the guidelines, and feel amazing. I have red wine, dark chocolate, and fruit as my main cheats. Outside of that, I try to keep the cheats to a minimum. I feel great though, and I'm never missing out. I had gone to the doctor several times for gut-related issues, but those are all gone now. I recently went to the doctor, and he was blown away by every test result. He laughed and quipped "Paleo must be working!" after reading through my numbers. It was a nice confirmation.

I ride my bike to work every day, about 4 miles round-trip. 3 times a week, I go to the local climbing gym to climb for an hour or so. I get to lift heavy things (me) and get a mental puzzle at the same time. It's an activity I can't recommend enough. I get to play in an adult playground, and get strong whilst doing so. Win/win.

I get made fun of here and there, but it's rare. The results sort of speak for themselves, and my family and friends have been pretty supportive. My mother is gluten intolerant, so is essentially Paleo as well. She lives nearby, so that makes things easy. Since I live in San Francisco, our culinary options are quite broad, which makes eating Paleo remarkably easy. In addition, most people here are aware of the Paleo lifestyle, and barely bat an eye at requests to lettuce-wrap or switch grains for veggies.

I'm energetic. I'm strong. I'm lean. I sleep well. I'm healthy, happy, quick, and ready to respond to anything life throws my way. Changing my diet, and ultimately my lifestyle, has allowed me the freedom to truly enjoy my life. I have no health issues, and have not gotten sick once since going Paleo. I feel that my body is primed to handle anything life can throw at it. I feel very grateful to the leaders of the Primal/Paleo movement, as they've been a great inspiration for me. I'd recommend the Paleo lifestyle to anyone I meet.

MARIE BENCIVENGA

SAN FRANCISCO, CALIFORNIA

mariebencivenga@gmail.com

Food has always been a serious part of my life. Growing up in an Italian household, many family traditions revolved around food – rich, indulgent, and often sugary foods that delighted my taste buds but affected me negatively weight-wise. I remember starting to worry about how my body looked around age 12, shortly after moving to the Los Angeles area. In the 8th grade I stopped growing taller and started to fill out. I went from a size 0 in 9th grade to a size 4 in 12th. I was involved in varsity sports in high school, but still had a soft belly and never felt very comfortable in my bikini, surrounded by all the beautiful valley girls. I also was plagued with allergies, asthma, and illnesses throughout childhood. My family always prepared meat, vegetables, and a starchy carb like potatoes, pasta, or rice with every dinner. I loved to snack on frozen meals, hot pockets, Del Taco, In 'n Out, and french fries, as well as dining out often and trying all the latest food fads. Still, at age 18, I was 5'3" and a healthy 118 pounds.

I moved to San Francisco after high school, and I got to thoroughly explore the city through its fabulous food. I spent long hours studying in architectural school, and survived on caffeine, pizza, and candy bars during projects. I gained the notorious "freshman fifteen" and continued to gain weight through sophomore year. I started to yo-yo between crash dieting and binge eating to reward myself for losing a few pounds. My waistline continued to grow during a semester abroad in Hungary. It was around this time that I stopped weighing myself and stopped caring. I was going to enjoy the flavors of all the foods I could try, and damn the consequences. I traveled Europe, experiencing every pastry I could along the way. I was always ill. My immune system didn't ever protect me, and I caught every cold that came along. I ate comfort foods to get better and eventually I came home from Europe wearing a size 8.

I continued to eat and crash diet, going between 130 and 150 pounds for the next few years. During that time I met Nick, my future husband. He had just moved to the city, and we spent a few years eating equal amounts of junk food and foodie fanfare. I also loved to cook by this time, and would make decadent chocolate trifles, baked peaches rolled in sugar and served with ice cream, blackberry cream butter crust pies, and more. We were stuck in this cycle of over-indulging, getting ill, eating junk to make ourselves "feel better" and then gaining more weight and starting over. Our exercise regimen had dissipated down to zero. We didn't like our jobs or our bodies. It was time for a change.

Nick and I accepted year-long teaching positions in Seoul, South Korea. We got engaged and I hated how I looked in the pictures we sent out to our family members. The day before the flight I weighed myself as I figured out the weight of my suitcase. I was 24, weighed 160 pounds, and was packing size 12 clothes to take with me. I was ashamed.

Upon arrival in Korea, I was bombarded with images of incredibly thin girls and surrounded by size 0 women. I would get waved away from stores when I entered, their broken English telling me, "No big size, no big size." After a young student openly mocked me in front of a class for my weight, I sat in my office and cried. I hated how I felt and how I looked. I was tired of always being sick and I wanted to change. My fiancé was on board.

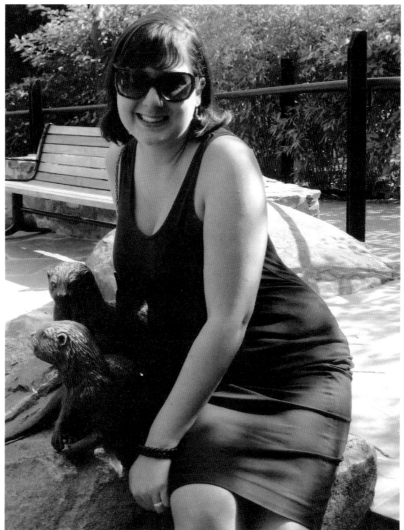

We were in the right place to start making a change. The Koreans eat lots of fermented food, meat, seasonal veggies, and rice. I decided early on during our contract that I would NOT be eating the rice served with every meal. I didn't know anything about grains or the science of food at this point. I only knew that rice made me feel extra full, and that I didn't want that feeling anymore. Culturally, bread and pasta aren't eaten as often in Korea as in the USA, so I essentially began to cut grains out of my diet. Nick and I cut back on sugars and ate lean meats and fresh veggies.

We decided to reintroduce exercise into our lives, and we chose the Insanity video program to try to help strengthen our bodies. The 60 day program helped me lose 15 pounds and two dress sizes. I felt good, but I wasn't where I wanted to be. Nick developed defined arms and the beginnings of a six pack. He was so excited. I started to feel left behind. We returned to the USA and I started to let my ego get the better of me. I was eating "healthy" but still had sugar and whole grains included in my diet. I was gaining some weight back and we were getting married soon. Right before we switched to the Primal lifestyle, I weighed around 140 pounds. A mistake had been made with my wedding dress alterations and it couldn't fit. I didn't know what I was going to do. I started to go through the Insanity program again, but I wanted something more. I didn't want to have to force myself to work out, I wanted to love exercising.

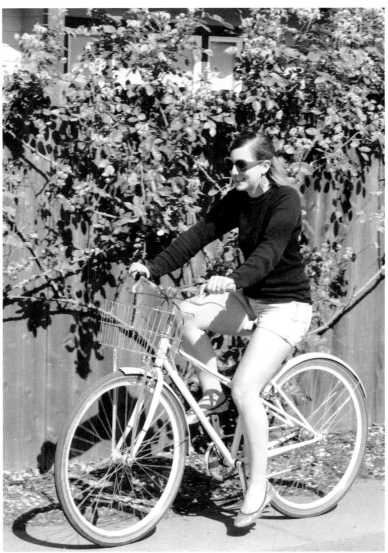

I found a local rock climbing gym and decided we were going to give it a shot. WE LOVED IT! We quickly signed up and began climbing indoors almost every night. This was right around the time that my fiancé was doing a lot of reading. He had found Gary Taubes' *Good Calories, Bad Calories,* and then been directed over to Mark's Daily Apple. He began to lecture me on our food choices and made powerful requests that we try a paleo lifestyle. While I couldn't really believe that all the conventional wisdom about food I believed in was wrong, I was eager to try anything and agreed to the 30 day trial.

The sugar and carb withdrawals were hard for me. I swear I smelled toast everywhere I went. But once that passed, I dropped a lot of weight really quickly. The 30 days raced by and we noticed a huge change in our sleep patterns, our mental clarity, and our digestive health; all for the better. We ate bacon every day, as well as fish, seasonal veggies from our CSA box, and plenty of cuts of meat. I cut out processed food and only bought organic or grass fed foods. Our bodies grew lean, as well as quite strong with all the climbing. By our wedding day, I weighed 123 pounds (at age 25) and felt amazing. All of our guests showered me with compliments and for the first time in a long time, I looked at photographs of myself and loved how I looked in every single one.

It has been almost two years of maintaining the paleo lifestyle. My husband is my life partner, my climbing partner, and my food partner. I have maintained my weight and still love the way I look and feel. Together we still climb around 3 times a week, ride our bicycles, lift heavy things sometimes, and walk all over our lovely (and hilly) city. My allergies and asthma are things of the past. I have only been sick twice during the entire time we've been paleo. My husband founded the Facebook SF Primal group and we have become a beautiful community of support and information. It is a constant source of inspiration and helps us stay on track. Our enthusiasm for the paleo lifestyle has helped several of our friends and family members also try the paleo path. We love the way we live and can't imagine going back.

KELLIE MORRILL

SEATTLE, WASHINGTON

www.evolvenatural.blogspot.com

I was the chubby kid who ate Hamburger Helper for dinner with soda. My single dad struggled to feed us healthy foods. I was 14 when I figured out that Corn Nuts and a Slurpee from the snack cart at school was cheaper than the meals I could purchase, and I could save the extra money to buy music CDs. This was also around the time I decided to become a vegetarian, despite my total lack of interest in vegetables. My diet for 14 years consisted mostly of pasta, cheese, and other white foods.

Fast forward 15 years, one baby and a failed marriage later, and I was exhausted, overweight and unhappy. Looking back, I believe that's when my adrenal glands really started to crash. I developed horrible acne, and my hair began to fall out. I tried every face cream on the market but it only got worse. I went to a dermatologist who put me on antibiotics and back onto hormonal birth control. When this didn't help, I finally went to a naturopath. She suggested I had Candida overgrowth, possible food allergies, WAY too much stress, was drinking too much caffeine, and I was not getting enough sleep. When I eliminated dairy from my diet I saw some improvements, but I wasn't satisfied.

I was a busy single mom relying heavily on packaged convenience food. I felt like a zombie and a hypocrite because the life I was living was not in line with my values, and I knew that I would feel better if I took the time to clean up my diet. I started reading about local economies and farmers markets and homesteading.

In 2011, I considered a detox or cleanse – but wasn't interested in starving myself. Then a friend encouraged me to try a whole-food paleo approach for 30 days and see how I felt. I began to eat simple, whole foods, as high quality as possible. I ate meat, eggs, nuts, fruits, vegetables, and oils. I ate when I was hungry, and stopped when I was full. I didn't measure or track anything. I ate fruit when I craved sweets.

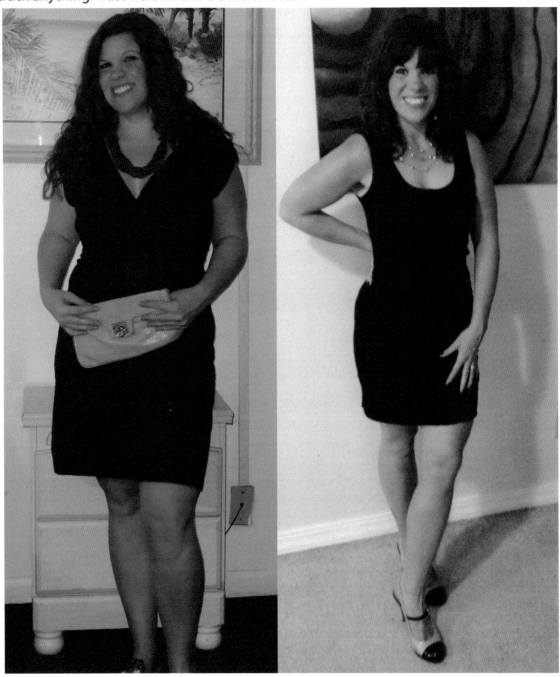

This is not some fad diet - it is a well-researched lifestyle change. I went for it and have NEVER looked back. I started with an average of three meals a day and a few snacks, but quickly noticed I very often wasn't hungry, and dropped snacks. I fell in love with the farmer's market and couldn't get enough new nutrition knowledge. I slowly added grass fed beef and pastured pork into my diet a couple of times a week.

I was inspired by the simple cooking recipes I found online and started to think this could be just what I need to learn to cook, support local economies, and improve my health all at once. I read Robb Wolf's *The Paleo Solution* from cover to cover and was fascinated by how much sense it all made. I began to understand the biochemistry of why my body felt the way it did, and how to fuel it properly. I learned how the government had come to endorse following a low-fat diet that kept the food and pharmaceutical companies rich, and the people sick and fat. I also got over my fear of healthy fats, after learning what "healthy fats" really meant. I learned to ignore most conventional nutrition wisdom, and really start thinking and learning for myself. This way of eating felt perfectly aligned with my values – and I never once worried about becoming another one of those annoying women who are always dieting or weighing themselves. Within two weeks my mental fog was gone, my skin was clearing, and I had boundless energy. The cravings faded away and I began to really enjoy cooking and eating real food.

Within a month of eliminating gluten and sugar, my son was having an easier time in school. When he was two years old, I eliminated dairy from his diet and his asthma and eczema went away completely. At age five, I had begun to slowly add dairy back into his diet. When I really started paying attention and understanding how food impacts mood, I realized that, although it no longer triggered his asthma, it made him feel emotionally out of control and clogged his sinuses. Without dairy and gluten he was more focused and more in control of his impulses and his emotions. It took a while to work up to a full change, but he now avoids sugar as well, and embraces healthy whole foods and snacks with enthusiasm.

In the first four months, I went from 185 pounds and size 14 to 145 pounds and a size 6, without much exercise at all - and without the obsessive diet brain. My skin was softer with a more even tone and fewer wrinkles. My hair was softer, growing in stronger than ever. I was cooking great meals, packing my lunches, and learning more every day about nutrition. I felt satisfied, and it got easier every day. In 6 months, I had more energy that I knew what to do with – so I started working out. I added walking and dancing to my routine a few nights a week, and tried crossfit and LOVED it. My weight began to shift again. I built muscle, lost inches, and dropped fat. A year and a half later, I'm down to a fit size 2. I lift weights and do high impact intensive training 2-3 times a week, and really enjoy pushing myself to be stronger and have more stamina. My mood and focus are fantastic!

My sister joined me and lost 30 pounds. My dad joined me and has lost over 20 pounds and reversed his type two diabetes. I'm still learning every day, and taking stock of my values. I've planted two gardens and a window herb box. I bought a juicer and I enjoy juicing greens in the morning. I'm having so much fun learning about nutrition and alternative health, I'm blogging all about it (evolvenatural.blogspot.com or find me on Facebook at Natural Evolution) and planning to go back to school and provide health coaching. I work with children with disabilities and meet kids every day who are struggling. I believe that a diet of whole foods that eliminates allergies can make a difference in everyone's lives. My dream is to help families of children with disabilities through holistic treatments that include diet interventions.

It's not always easy making big changes, but I've never regretted putting myself first and making positive changes for my own health and wellbeing. I've connected with my local community and I can honestly say I can't remember the last time I bought a Coke, Nestle, or Monsanto product. I have joined a local produce buyers club, become a regular at the farmers market, joined a CSA at a neighborhood farm that also donates to my son's school, and even joined in with friends to pool our money together to buy a ¼ cow from a local butcher. I swap and share fish and veggies with my neighbors and barter work exchanges. I'm so much happier, healthier, and closer to my dreams than I ever thought I could be, in just one short year.

SOPHIE LUCAS

MONTREAL, CANADA

www.youtube.com/getbackinshape

I was a very active kid. I loved to play many sports. I was always the first girl picked on all the team sports at school because I was one of the best. I had inherited my mother's genes for being very slim, but my dad's side is another story. When I turned 10, I was hit with a hip growth sickness, because I had grown too fast. I had to have two surgeries and that left me completely inactive for two years while recovering. In those two years, all I had to do was eat. During that time, I gained a lot of fat that I was to later struggle with for many years…up until a few years ago. I had become obese, and some would even say morbidly obese because I was tipping the scale at nearly 275 pounds at one point.

I can't say that I was unhappy though, because I was not. Of course I had those "I am fat" crisis moments, but I was still very active and played a lot of sports. I even played elite competitive softball for twelve years. I had boyfriends and a great social life. I felt good inside - but I was always "How do I look under all that fat?" People have the misconception - and even go as far as saying to bigger people - "Oh, well, you have big bones." Yeah right. I can definitely tell you right now that I do not have big bones.

So what finally motivated me to lose all that weight? Well I can honestly say that there were a few motivating factors: (1) the birth of my daughter. I wanted to be a great example for her and I wanted her to be proud of me; (2) my constant wondering to see how I looked under all that fat. Why couldn't I look as good as I felt most of the time? There was someone I knew I would love under there, and I desperately wanted to see her; and (3) my endless health problems that kept getting worse and worse as time went on.

I have heart burn that turned into terrible acid reflux, heart palpitations, joint pain, tiredness, gas - so much gas from both ends, lack of energy, and just overall a bad feeling about my long term health.

My journey began in August of 2003. It was far from easy, but with all the great help and support I got from the people at my gym, my family, and my friends I managed to lose 100 pounds in twelve months - going from 250 pounds to 150 pounds. My motto "Do not give in to failure" was my inspiration and was given to me by a great trainer and spinning instructor Vincent Kuziomko. As if losing all the weight wasn't enough, in April of 2004 I decided I needed new goals to motivate me in my training. So I took on the new challenge of completing a triathlon which I did. Then I started training for fitness competitions, competing for three years. I also competed in the Canadian finals of the 2007 Miss Hawaiian Tropic.

My diet was personalized from week to week in accordance with my training and my own personal macronutrient needs (protein, carbs, and essentials fats). My training program was designed on a twelve month cycle and was further personalized depending on my progress, strength, and weaknesses. I worked out three times a week and did cardio three times a week as well. I ate healthy, in a non-paleo way, back then: Lots of low fat, artificial sweeteners, transformed foods. Although it wasn't paleo, it was a big step in the right direction from what I had been eating before.

If I would have known that what I did back then to lose the weight would have the effect that I had to deal with NOW, in 2012, I would have gone about it completely differently.

In late 2007, I felt very ill for several months. I was diagnosed with "over training." I had trouble sleeping. I was tired all the time. I couldn't train anymore at all. This went on for about five months, and in those five months, I gained back about 60 pounds. When I was finally better, I tried to get back into the gym, but as soon I as I did, my body would send me distress signals and I would have to stop. I slowly went back to my bad eating habit to comfort me, and in the next two years went all the way back to 240 pounds. With that came back all my awful health symptoms that had all completely disappeared with my prior weight loss. And I was depressed. In those two years I must have tried to get back on the health saddle about TWENTY times, abandoning it each time after two or three weeks.

On January 1, 2010 I joined the YouTube weight loss community and started v-logging. For some reason, this helped me rediscover my motivation and consistency. And after a few weeks, my body finally started to show signs of weight loss…but not without hardship. The years of bad eating, being obese, the weight loss, the harsh training, and fitness competitions all came back to haunt me: I was diagnosed with a herniated disk that kept me from working out. Despite this, I was determined and I stuck to my eating plan - and for the first time in my entire life, I lost weight, without exercising, only through food. I was so happy.

The year after, I had finally recovered from my back injury and I started training again. This time I was hit once with a neck hernia caused by a neck injury I had sustained while doing a fitness competition. So there I was again, not able to train, and in the chiropractor's office a few times a month. But once again I refused to give up, and I kept on losing weight. After two years I was down about 30 pounds and I was happy - but all my health troubles remained and the weight loss did nothing for them this time around. I had heart burn again, acid reflux, heart palpitations, trouble sleeping, anxiety, panic attacks, lots of gas, stomach pain, and joint pain - like the kind of pain you get after a marathon - except I hadn't run one. Why was I still so sick, even if I was losing the weight?!? I was starting to get scared.

In February 2012, I was still having so many health issues. I talked to a good friend of mine who introduced me to his world of paleo - a lifestyle. I was immediately curious. When we met and he told me all about it, I felt like I just finally found what I had been looking for all this time. I believe if someone had told me about paleo a long time ago, I might not have been able to do it. I was so stuck in my ways of fake sugar and low fat I would never have believed it. But after all my successes and failures, I embraced it completely and dove in head first. In the back of my head I have always kind of known this was the way to go. I mean how can

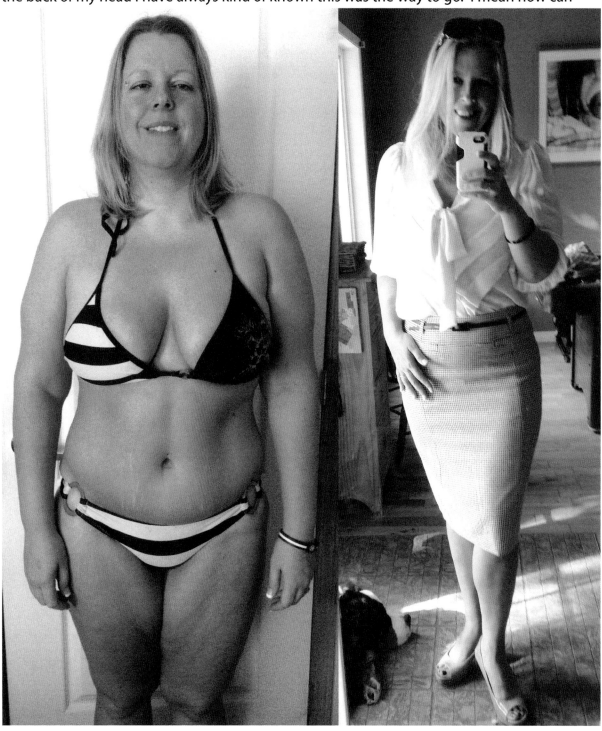

someone go wrong eating 100% unprocessed foods consisting of vegetables, fruits, meats, nuts and good fats? They can't. So I started with the Whole30 program and it was unlike anything I had ever experienced. The first two to three weeks were hard, very hard. I felt depressed, weak, and all sorts of weird stuff - but with the help of my friend who kept checking up on me and explaining that it was my body withdrawing from excess carbs. He said it would all be better in a few weeks, so I kept at it, if only to discover what was on the other side. Next thing I know I felt magnificent. I felt like a new woman. All my health symptoms were fading away, and for a few weeks, I was in heaven - then another setback happened.

As I started eating more and more healthy fats, I suddenly started having a lot of problem digesting them, and was experiencing severe pains that would last for hours, waking up in the middle of the night with such sharp attacks that I would end up in the emergency room. After much testing, I was diagnose with gall bladder stones. Remember I said "I knew then what I know now"? Well this is it. My stones we caused by a few different factors: bad eating for most of my life, the rapid weight loss, then eating low fat.

Eating low fat is not the answer to anything. By adopting a healthy paleo lifestyle, the fat was actually triggering my attacks. I was desperate. I was told I needed surgery to have my gall bladder removed. I was so upset and did not want to do it.

After much research and the help of my friends and family and many people in the IMPG Facebook group (http://is.gd/paleogroup) I decided to try to cure myself naturally and underwent eight weeks of natural treatment, including stone flushes. It was HELL. Eight weeks of eating 100% vegetarian, and almost 100% of it raw, so that my body could cleanse itself and alkaline as much as possible. Once I did this, and I felt 100 times better. After another scan, I still have some stones, but I could feel my body functioning a lot better. I could again digest fats. I haven't had an attack ever since.

I am now 37 years old, 5'9", and I weigh 180 pounds. When I started paleo, on February 1, 2012, I was 205 pounds. Since going paleo, I switched everything about the way I eat. I now only eat non processed foods and almost 100% organic. I have nine of my own chickens now and can eat pastured eggs. I grow my own fresh veggies and I have planted several fruit trees. A former meal for me would have been two slices of whole wheat bread with light peanut butter and sugar free strawberry jam and a huge glass of milk and orange juice. During the day I would have so much Crystal Light juice…in retrospect it is impossible to believe the amount of toxins I was drinking. A treat for me would have been a meal at a restaurant, like pasta, drinks, and of course something chocolate for dessert. Now for me, a treat is some apples dipped in macadamia nut butter and maple syrup sauce. You should try it, it's so good!

My husband and daughter have been supportive, although not as much I would like. I have decided that this is all about me, and I can lead by example, and I refuse to feel guilty for someone else's choices. As for my daughter, I am making changes to her habits slowly, and I think in time she will too see all the health benefits. What ten-year-old says she hates McDonald's because it makes her tummy hurt? Well I am quite happy to say that mine does. She hasn't had McDonald's in over eight months!

What pleases me the most about my new lifestyle is that feeling I get when I sit, in front of a meal consisting of eggs I gathered myself that morning, salads and veggies I collected in my garden. And when I eat, I know, I KNOW, that I am finally doing what every human being should be doing: giving their body what it truly deserves: The best. And now that's how I try to live my life, putting myself first, giving myself only what is best for me - because I know if I don't do it, no one else will. I only have one life and I want to live it, as best as I possibly can. For me, eating that meal is probably how someone else feels when they buy $10,000 worth of mags for their Mercedes Benz…only the best! Guess which one of us has it right?

I would like to end with this: When did the human life become so unimportant? We treat our cars, our homes, even our freakin' animals better then we treat ourselves. The government and the big corporations have become so insatiable wanting more and more money that our lives have become expendable, secondary to their profits. If we do not take action, we will just die a slow painful death.

JOSEPH SALAMA

SAN RAFAEL, CALIFORNIA

joe@salama.com

Throughout my life, I had food allergies, seasonal allergies, and I used to get food stuck in my throat (past the epiglottis, I could still breathe) and would not be able to eat any more until I dislodged the food, often times a noisy, violent, and socially-inappropriate process.

I was always an excellent student, I high school and in college. I had perfected the ability to cram effectively and still get one of the top grades. When I went to law school however, something started to gradually change. I was no longer able to focus as well as before. I found that regular exercise helped counteract this. I co-founded a running club on campus, really got into running, and set my one and two mile PRs (5:09 and 10:55) on the same day. Although exercise helped me focus, something was still wrong. My grades were not as high as before, and I was having trouble organizing my work and getting it done.

Also, oddly, I noticed I couldn't hear as well from my right ear. I figured it was from going to too many concerts and from blasting my car stereo too much in my youth. Plus I was getting a little older, and my body was bound to stop working perfectly at some point. Made sense to me.

After I graduated from law school, I got involved with Team In Training, a fantastic organization that is dedicated to raising money for blood cancer research. I eventually completed 5 marathons and 9 half marathons around the world. I loved running. It became very meditative and therapeutic for me. At the same time, my ability to focus was getting worse and worse, and I had trouble holding jobs. I was always enthusiastic and eager, and tried really hard, but for some reason it wasn't working. My attention to detail seemed to be slipping, and so was my ability to plan projects and estimate the amount of time it would take to complete them.

About 7 years ago, I went to see a psychopharmacologist who tested me for everything under the sun, finally concluding that I had ADHD. His diagnosis was confirmed by another physician. He was an extremely intelligent physician with extraordinary credentials from excellent institutions. He prescribed Vyvanse to me (an amphetamine, a longer-lasting Adderall), and told me that with it came an education. He was determined to try to get me to understand why I had ADHD to enable me to better cope with it. He told me that ADHD is genetic. He told me that I was genetically designed to be a hunter, and because I was forced to live in a modern world, my brain had trouble adapting. I could look back on this and laugh at the irony of it, but it's not funny when you are paying thousands of dollars for treatment of something when a short discussion about diet could have returned me to the way I used to be in a matter of weeks.

But ADHD is not curable! It's genetic! There is no cure! You have to learn to live with it! And so I did – as much as anyone can learn to live with it. The medication and regular exercise certainly helped me focus a lot more, and enabled me to start my own legal practice with success.

About three years ago, I began to devote a lot of time and energy to self-improvement. I learned a lot about psychology, gender communication issues, and parenting (by then I had two gorgeous children, Mark and Amira, my muses). A good friend of mine named David Storey "casually" mentioned to me – about 8 or 9 times – to try "going paleo," stating that I would reap a lot of benefit from it. I didn't really have any idea what paleo was, but in the interest of self-improvement, I gave it a try.

The next 2.5 weeks of carb flu were extremely difficult. I USED TO LIVE ON GRAINS. Although paleo is not a low carb diet, simply cutting the grains from your diet will result in a much lower carb intake – and you just might have the same carb flu I did.

During this time, I started listening to a Gary Taubes' *Good Calories, Bad Calories* which I downloaded from audible.com (thanks to Shirley McLean for the recommendation!), a 600 page/25+ hour book. As my brain was fogged from the carb flu, I heard countless hours of studies and research that concluded that grains were to blame for countless diseases, everything from heart disease to Alzheimer's. By the time I was ¼ of the way in, I was sold. I was disgusted by grains. I knew that this change was going to be permanent.

About 2.5 weeks in, I looked at my work calendar and noticed I had a deadline coming up – the very next day in fact. I am a lawyer and had to oppose a motion. I got a good night's sleep to try to get the fog to lift a bit, and woke up feeling a lot closer to normal. I started reading the legal papers I had to respond to at about 9:30 a.m. There were two inches of papers to review. By 10:20, I finished and started writing my responsive papers. At 11:45 I finished what I thought was a thorough and persuasive response. I looked at the page count, and I was only five pages! Pretty short. I reviewed everything all over again just to be sure – when you have ADHD you learn to check your work. Everything checked out…except I thought it was a little redundant. So I edited it down to four pages. Four pages to oppose about 100 pages. But I was sure. So I sent it to the court by fax, and looked at the clock – it was only 1:00 p.m.! I thought to myself the same thing I thought after every other big project

I had done the 6 years before, "Thank goodness for the ADHD medication or I would not have been able to focus like that." Then it hit me: I didn't take my ADHD medication that day! I vowed to never pump my body full of medicine ever again. And when the judge quoted my papers, ruling in favor of my client, that sealed the deal.

I have since been officially diagnosed as not having ADHD. I can organize, plan, orchestrate, linger, listen, focus, and relax with the best of them. And I no longer have the desire to compete in endurance events in order to seek peace from the extra stimulation. And my law and mediation practice has become that much more successful. I still believe that ADHD is genetic, but I think it would be more accurate to say that an ADHD response to eating grains is genetic. And I may not officially have "cured" it, but there are no symptoms until and unless I eat grains.

Obviously, I was a bit upset by this. I was upset that neither of my doctors told me anything about diet and the importance of diet in dealing with ADHD. I have no doubt that they are up on the latest information – it is just that the latest information doesn't include anything about nutrition. As you will see in other stories in this book, the mainstream medical community is all about treatment of symptoms through drugs, not addressing the underlying source of the problem.

The irony of course is that my doctor told me that I was designed to live in a cave and hunt – but failed to consider that if that were true, my body would be genetically adopted to eating Paleolithic/pre-agricultural foods, rather than a SAD/post-agricultural diet consisting in large

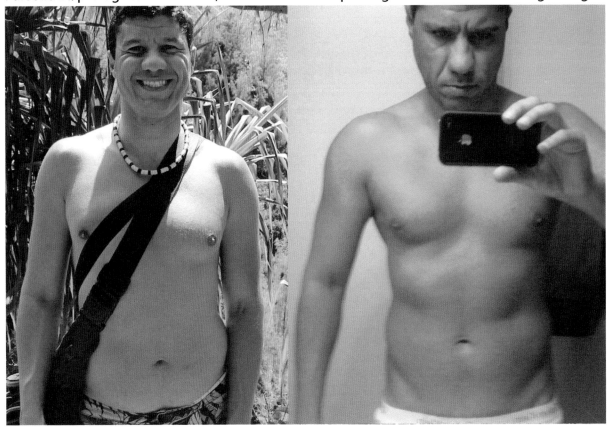

part of processed grains.

My food allergies, seasonal allergies, eating problem, and hearing problem are all gone. I have more energy than ever, and feel 15 years younger. And as a side bonus, something I had never considered, my body composition has changed with almost no effort. In the photo on the left, I was running half and full marathons and eating a SAD diet. In the photo on the right, I was exercising a mere 90 minutes a week, but eating paleo. This transformation happened in 4 months.

I also got my parents doing paleo too. My mom's type II diabetes is much more under control, and she rarely checks her blood glucose levels anymore. My 80-year old father had been fighting Parkinson's for over a decade when I introduced him to paleo. He was eating a lot of processed foods, in addition to the whole grains. His doctors at UCSF Neurology – all of whom I have no doubt are brilliant at what they do – told him that there would be no improvement, and that it's simply a question of how fast his brain deteriorates. After one week on paleo, no processed foods, grains, legumes, or dairy, he became far more lucid and engaged than he had been over the prior 6 months. He was now able to get himself out of his chair and out of bed almost every time he tried. He's more sociable and happier. It is nothing short of a miracle that for the first time in the last ten years, his condition has actually improved - dramatically. After three weeks, he lost weight and had more energy. His dementia has disappeared, his nightmares disappeared, and they have stayed that way.

I now have well over 80 converts under my belt. And like everyone who does paleo, I feel like I have been given a new life. That is why I am so enthusiastic about it and decided to compile this book. I know that part of my mission in life is to help others see that there is an alternative to eating whole grains, working out like crazy, and not having the body you want. And on the medical side, there might just be an alternative to all those prescriptions and dollars. I hope that someone reading this will take a second look at their situation and make a change for the better. Life is too short to be poisoning yourself with food and be far below your potential, and not even know it.

KLAUS JESPERSEN

BUDAPEST, HUNGARY

kj@cavemensfood.com , www.cavemensfood.com , http://is.gd/cavemensfood

I have always been active in sports, and have held had 2- 3 jobs ever since I was 11. I was never really sick, and never had any problem with my weight. I used to always eat many huge meals, and was raised to fear high dietary fat, and was always told carbohydrates are fine. And as long as I was young and active, there was no problem. Although I never made to the national competition level, I played a lot of different sports: soccer, basketball, squash, badminton, table tennis, running, coaching at a fitness club, skiing, biking, and roller-skating. I was never on any prescription medicine, never smoked, and never liked sodas. I always felt strong and healthy.

Things started to change as I got into my 30s. I became less active, started driving instead of biking, and started a family. I moved and started commuting instead of working out. Even though I did a lot less activity, my appetite did not go down, and because I was eating low fat high carb foods, I felt safe.

I was slowly gaining weight – 2 pounds every 6 months. It was so gradual that I didn't notice too much. At 6', 1" tall and broad shouldered, I did not appear overweight. I used to have a lot of excess gas and never knew why.

My basic diet (before paleo) was meat with pasta, potato and bread, rye bread - which everybody in Scandinavia thinks is much healthier than white bread. I always loved meat and never felt full, or good, without it. I now wonder why I didn't listen to my body back then. I remember one time on a Saturday morning in 2006, we made some fresh bread with homemade jam and I found myself two hours later driving on the road, shaking, not knowing what was going on. Once I realized that my breakfast had been just empty fast carbs, I knew that something was wrong with my diet.

In 2008 I was newly divorced, and had a chance to see things from a new perspective. I realized my health was a mess. I was fat and had low energy. I knew I needed to make a change. I decided to start running, and on my first day, after less than 5 minutes, I was nearly dying, unable to even jog home. What happened to the fit me?

In March 2008 I signed up with a running club, and my goal was to complete a half marathon and lose 22 pounds. I was just over 200 pounds at the time. In 6 months, I managed to lose 13 pounds, and completed a half marathon with a decent time. A few weeks after the race, I had a leg injury because I was running too much for my body to handle. I lost motivation and gained back all the weight I lost, plus more, setting a new personal record. In 2009 I reached 231 pounds, and was too heavy to run.

At the start of 2010, a very good friend of mine suggested I look into CrossFit. CrossFit was completely unknown to me, and I got in to it slowly, doing calisthenics on my own rather than at a gym. I LOVED IT. I got an incredible workout and was done in 20-40 minutes. I started to add some weight to my workouts, and read up on CrossFit and watched a lot of videos online. I was fascinated with it.

That same friend came back from a CrossFit certification class and told me to sign up because it "will give you a lot of inspiration." So I signed up. I was given materials, and I looked them over. It was there that I first read about paleo. "Food is medicine" it read. I was intrigued and had to check it out.

I was not in very good shape compared to the rest of the guys at the seminar. I was older and bigger at 220 pounds. Coming back from the seminar fully motivated, I cut all grains, potato, rice, and all fast food out of my diet. I also stepped up my CrossFit training. In just a few months, I lost ten pounds. It was a big day for me. I felt as if I did not really have to fight that hard for it – so I decided to set another goal of losing another ten pounds – something that I would have considered completely unrealistic just six months before.

On May 10, 2011, I weighed in at just under 187 pounds! It was an AWESOME DAY! I was gaining muscle too, which weighs more than fat, and I looked great! I was now the same weight I was at 20 years old, 25 years before.

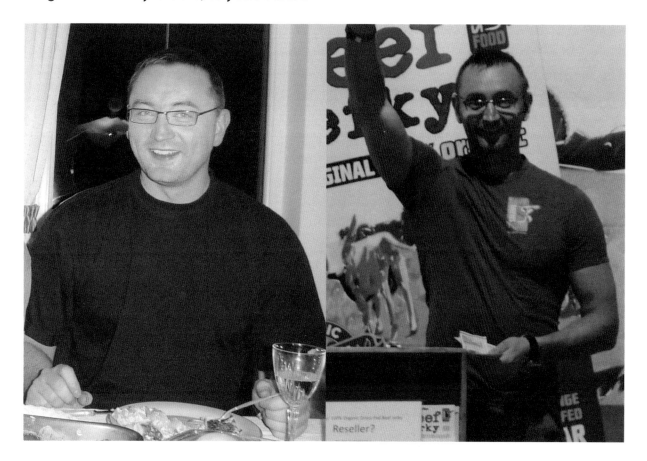

At first my girlfriend and my daughter did not really enjoy my paleo "trip." But I was often the cook, and they accepted what I served them. Sometimes they added pasta, potatoes, or other other non paleo foods, but not as much as before. After a while they got fed up (or maybe they wised up?) by my commentary "Why do you eat that shit?" and started eating less and less of it. Now they are both 98% paleo at home.

In the summer of 2011, I got a shock when Anna (my then 12 year old daughter) came home after 3 weeks alone with her grandmother: she gained 11 pounds in 3 weeks! She had acne on her face which she never had before, was lethargic, and looked very unhealthy overall. She told me why: She ate bread for breakfast, cake, waffles, candy, chips, and sodas. All served with love by her grandmother. I was in horror.

We agreed that if Anna ate what I suggested for 4 weeks, she would get the biggest ice cream in town. She ate paleo for 4 weeks and was in good spirits about it. She lost 9 pounds, lost her acne, had more energy, and got her positive attitude back. She asked me "Papa, if I continue, can I get a little potato along the meat and greens every two weeks?" She got a deal. ☺

Food IS medicine. I had a small spot of eczema on my leg that grew and shrank over time, and sometime spread to my elbow and forehead. My dermatologist gave me some cream for it, and it worked – for two weeks – after which time it returned. When I called her back, I told her that I did not want to use the cream but find the cause of the problem. She replied: "Sorry I can't help you, there can be endless reasons for this." After these 18 months, I decided to get tested for everything under the sun. I was told "you are in the same condition as a young strong athlete." All the while, my eczema keep growing, itching, and becoming damn ugly. I eventually discovered I was deficient in omega 3 fatty acids. So now I eat fish or take fish oil supplements. Food is medicine. When you eat and drink you either feed disease or fight it.

Without doubt I can say CrossFit and paleo changed my life BIG TIME. I found out it was hard to be paleo and travel, and was trying to figure out how to get my hands on beef jerky – which was perfect for traveling.

I imagined other paleo people have the same problem, so I started to make my own brand, which you can find here: www.cavemensfood.com. I sell 100% Organic Grass-Fed Beef Jerky in 4 flavors. I launched my business at the CrossFit Regionals in Copenhagen in May 2012 and it was a huge success. I almost have more business than I can handle!

It is now September of 2012. I am 46 years old, and weigh 187 pounds and am in the best shape of my life!

CAROL LOVETT

SIMCOE, ONTARIO, CANADA

ditchthewheat@gmail.com , www.ditchthewheat.com

Before I changed my diet, my life was out of control. I was feeling dizzy, my stomach was in agony, and my headaches had been an everyday nuisance since high school. I started noticing I had episodes of dizziness when I was working in my first job after college in an accounting department. The simple task of leaving my desk to walk to the photocopier was becoming a struggle. The room was spinning, I could not walk straight. I incurred numerous episodes of vertigo for many years but they would happen quickly and disappear for months. Like any health problem, I brushed it off and went on with my life.

The recession started, and I made the decision to continue my education. I gave my notice at work and pursued my degree in Business Commerce, in Toronto, Canada. My first year back in school after working full time for a few years was hard. I was older, but still young at 24 years. Right after I started the year, I immediately gained the "freshman fifteen", which lead to a total of 30 pounds in less than 6 months. I was eating pizza and calzones in between classes. Soon my bothersome dizziness came back with a vengeance.

I could no longer do normal things. The vertigo episodes took over my new life as a student. I could barely walk around the mall without sitting every five minutes. The attacks would happen while I was standing, sitting, lying down, or waking up from a night's rest. I could no longer focus on school work or in class. My turning point happened when I was watching *Mystery Diagnosis*. I eagerly watched as a similar story unfolded on the screen. Within a week I called my doctor, set up an appointment and faced my medical dilemma head on. I was referred to an internal specialist.

I twitched and I squirmed as I sat uncomfortably in the chair in front of the specialist. He grilled me on how I felt, my vertigo experiences, my stomach pains, and my headaches. He poked and prodded me until I was exhausted. After a few visits he prescribed me Serc pills, to be taken 4 times a day, to treat vertigo. Finally, after a few months of weekly visits, brain scans, blood tests, I heard the words leave his mouth "I am diagnosing you with Meniere's Disease." I was happy but upset. On the one hand, we knew what was going on, but on the other, I was in my mid twenties and I already had a disease. My specialist did not wait long before diving into another issue, my ballooning weight.

I started my clean-eating journey a week before Christmas. I was sitting in my doctor's office and he told me for the third time that I had to start losing weight. This time was different. I explained to him once again that I had tried and I was exercising. I was eating whole-wheat wraps instead of regular bread. I thought "What more could he ask for?!?" He finally exclaimed "Ditch the wheat!" That week I committed myself to a wheat-free diet.

I was a week into my new lifestyle. My doctor's orders were to eat zero wheat and reduce my carbs. Ok, sounds easy but I was lost. How do you eat lunch if it's not a sandwich? Which t.v. dinners are good for me? I was finishing my Christmas shopping and I stumbled into a thrift store. I often explored thrift stores since I love finding unique vintage items. I made my way over to the book section. I was glancing over all the health book titles as I saw an Atkins diet book. I grabbed it and thought *'this is a low carb diet that avoids wheat.'* I quickly flipped through it and felt this is going to be my guideline. I bought the book for a staggering one dollar and left the store ready to embark on my journey.

The Atkins diet emphasizes 4 phases. The first phase is a detox phase, Phase 1 tests different food categories, Phase 2 teaches you to find your carbohydrate tolerance for maintaining your weight loss, finally Phase 3 is maintenance. I felt very confident using the Atkins diet to fulfill my doctor's wishes. Everything went smoothly.

I transitioned during a weird time. The holidays are filled with binging and party after party. I stood alone in a room full of family and friends starring at the food. "Is this gluten free?" I found myself asking over and over again. "How did you prepare this? Was there flour involved in making this sauce?" Luckily parties are usually buffets, as opposed to sit-down dinners. Navigating through the buffet was easier than I expected. I grabbed deli meats, shrimp, cheese, veggies, and fruit. I nibbled away at my "rabbit food" as some people called it. I looked away when people stared and asked "are you crazy? Why are you avoiding wheat, of all things? Don't you know wheat is essential to an everyday diet?" Day after day of eating a wheat free diet I felt great. As crazy as it sounds, I started a diet during the holidays – and I actually enjoyed it!

I visited my specialist about four weeks later. I bounced into his office, gleaming, look at me! He noticed immediately I had lost weight, roughly fifteen pounds. Then I turned to him and said, "not only did I lose weight but my headaches reduced, my vertigo became better, and my stomach pains completely disappeared." The visits to the doctor's office became easier and easier as I felt better.

The Atkins diet encourages you to test food groups, such as dairy. I found early on, dairy didn't like me. I refused to give up on it. I loved cheese, and above else I loved cheesecake. I found myself leaning towards paleo recipes because I felt better not eating dairy. As I read paleo-inspired blogs and books I found myself questioning the food I ate and how it affected my body. I went beyond considering how wheat affected me and gained a lifestyle. A lifestyle that involved eating real food. I switched from my beloved sweeteners and used real honey and maple syrup to sweeten desserts. I found myself questioning the shampoo, make-up, and deodorant I placed on my body. I became concerned with where my food came from

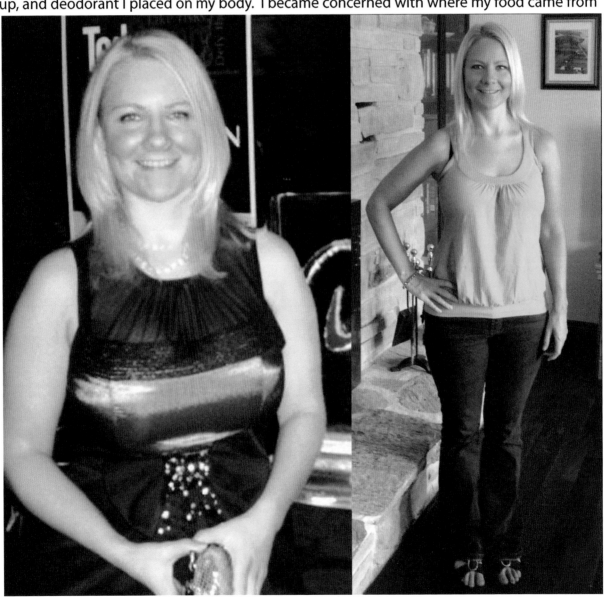

and how it was made. I sourced local grass fed beef and I visited the farm that the beef were raised on. I had a new relationship and respect for food and the environment. I became *paleo*, and I lost thirty pounds.

S. K.

ROCKLAND COUNTY, NEW YORK

I am a 50 year old woman and am currently en route overseas to meet my newest grandchildren (newborn babies and cousins #s 5 and 6 grandchildren)! It's totally remarkable what life brings if we allow ourselves to feel and learn.

A few short years ago I was scared out of my mind. I was considered obese and had lived through far too many medical diagnoses that were really, really intense and threatening. Cancer, diabetes, high cholesterol were all new to me, and I wanted none of them. I needed to change but was truly stumped.

Was it in my genes or was I doing it to myself? My Dad had died of cancer a few years prior, yet had also struggled with heart disease and high cholesterol. My older sister also had had a miserable time fighting cancer. My brother had high cholesterol and a major heart attack before the age of 50 – and he is slim and (we thought) fit. Even my Mom had her bout with cancer years ago, and has low blood pressure to boot! Talk about "high risk"!

During my last 20 some years, I had been vegetarian for 14 of them, and have tried raw foods, veganism, macrobiotics, and all the variations thereof. I was raised by Mom to love and appreciate food and have found a passion (as did she) in being a chef. I have always tried to provide good, clean wholesome food to my family and friends. Over the years, I think I may have tried every possible meal plan except that of the caveman.

Somewhere along the way, my weight escalated to 225 pounds. I started exercising, and tried doing yoga, swimming, aerobics, playing tennis, working out with a trainer, pilates, and many other things. These were all done for reasonable periods of time, but I never felt compelled to continue them – I was never satisfied with the results. I was also busy raising a family with four beautiful children. I had dropped out of high school to marry. Eventually, when my youngest was in preschool, I decided to go to college and get a formal education. At that point, I had a lot of commitments – and they only increased when I started my graduate work and internship. It was clear that something had to give - and more often than not, it was my motivation and time spent trying to change my appearance.

But when disease finally came knocking at my door, I was forced to recommit to changing my physique and becoming the healthiest person I could be. After all, I wanted to be around for a long time to enjoy my family and to meet my grandchildren.

I decided to pursue yoga more diligently and become a yoga instructor. During my training in July 2006, one of my teachers, Keith, was wearing a CrossFit t-shirt. I had developed a nice rapport with him at the time and he offered me an opportunity "to really see what fitness was all about." At the time, I had never seen people working out the way crossfitters did, and I thought they were lunatics. After witnessing that, I left in a hurry and had a hard time facing him a day or two later. I thought he was a total nutcase, and I finally told him that there is no way in hell I would ever do what they were doing.

Well next thing I know, after several months of private work, I actually started crossfitting. Keith introduced me to The Zone Diet. By then, I had tried so many ways of eating, and was appalled at his insistence that I needed to eat meat to become strong. I just couldn't do it after going so long without it.

Well one day, on my own, I went to a favorite restaurant and ordered grilled chicken breast.

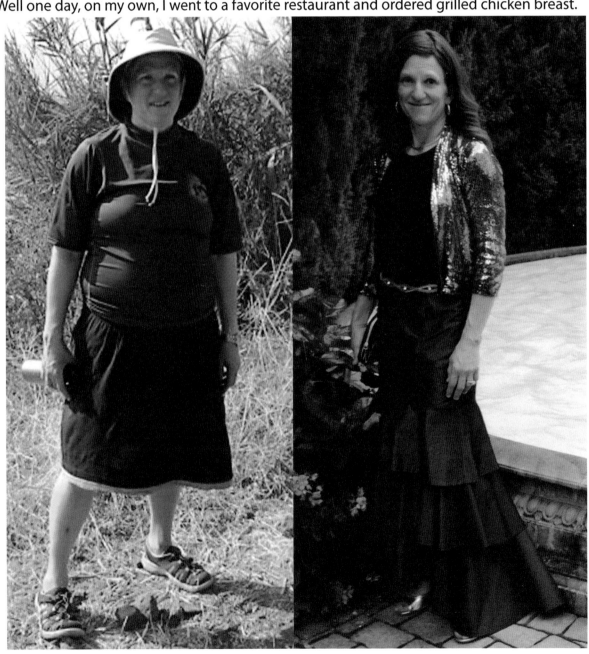

The server, who knew me, looked at me and asked if I was sure I wanted to eat meat. I haven't looked back since. Slowly I learned how to manage the macronutrients of the Zone eating plan. I started losing weight and gaining muscle. Keith insisted I eat a 1 block snack a half hour before every training session. This amounted to half an apple, 3 almonds and 1 hard-boiled egg. He had me eating a total of 10 blocks daily. I had already been eating organic, natural foods and now strived to add the best quality meat possible too... not an easy feat when you are strictly Kosher too!

A few years have since passed and life has handed me more trials and yet many more happy occasions. I am now certified as a Crossfit instructor, an Olympic Weightlifting coach and learning and adhering to the principals of paleo eating to a capital T! I have stopped making excuses about the cards I was dealt "genetically" or otherwise, have recommitted, and completely turned my life around.

I now train five days a week and am in the best shape I have ever been in...lean and fit. My body fat is excellent and low. I now compete in Olympic Weightlifting and have even won a few medals! I am totally committed to working with my coach and while he is tough, I really must thank him for all the lessons (even the painful ones) he has taught me, both in the gym and in LIFE! In addition, paleo is now my life and following its course means keeping my health. Plus, my health has created a business niche for me as a chef providing paleo meals for others.

So my question to you is: How do you want to feel as you get older?

I can't actually reverse the clock but I can sure as hell do my utmost to enjoy the days I walk this earth with health, commitment, and dignity…or as my coach, Coach Ray, says, with "sniper focus!"

HOWARD SMOOT

FARMERS BRANCH, TEXAS

I was overweight most of my adult life. At one point I was up to about 265 pounds, and I am 5', 11" tall. I ate mostly a standard American diet of processed foods with plenty of refined carbs. I was fat and miserable. I knew something had to change. My big sister, Jan (check out her awesome site: www.janssushibar.com) played a big part I my changes because she and my brother-in-law had just begun a real food approach to life just a few months earlier. They sent me a copy of "Fat Head" the movie. That movie jarred me. I highly recommend it to anyone who currently eats a SAD diet, and wants to lose weight and/or reclaim their life back.

The change started slowly at first, eliminating all refined carbs and sweets (bread, crackers, chips, cookies, cakes, candy, ice cream, etc.). After a couple of months, enthusiastic about the weight melting off, we spent a lot of time online and learned more about healthy food. We started getting our meat from local farms (grassfed meat) as well as eggs, milk, cheeses, and vegetables. All organic, local, pastured. Even today, almost two years into it, we are refining things, and are adding in some fermented foods like Kimchi and Kombucha for good gut bacteria.

My loving wife was signed on 100% from the get go. I applaud her, and highly recommend spouses make the change together. Personally, I think it is a deal maker, or breaker. At first my wife and I just wanted to lose weight. But after reading so much material online during the first year, we learned about the health benefits of eating paleo. Then we started on the kids. One processed grain product at a time, we gradually got these kids eating mostly real food (for the first time in their lives!). The health of our family improved right before our eyes. My children and my wife are really all I have. It turned out to be so much bigger than just losing weight.

I was not expecting anything other than weight loss, but boy did I get a LOT of surprises! Within TWO WEEKS my chronic daily heartburn had vanished completely. Poof! Just like that. I had been taking heartburn pills every single day for several years. And I haven't bought those little bastards in almost 2 years now. Then, I noticed my severe sleep apnea had stopped. I asked my wife if she'd noticed it, and she said I don't even snore anymore!

About two years before going grain free, I started getting what I called "broken glass" vision. Out of nowhere, I'd get these lines appearing in my vision that seemed like I was looking through broken glasses. It would take about 5 minutes to go away, and it happened maybe once per week for about 2 years. I haven't had that since going paleo. Also starting about 2 years before going paleo, I was losing my voice on a pretty regular basis for no 'reason' at all – this happened about 4 times per year with no other symptoms. I haven't had that happen since going paleo either.

Other than LOVING the way I look now, I also feel so FANTASTIC. Every day is a gift that I look forward to. Where as before…well, not so much.

Before paleo I did a "Tae Bo" cardio routine, about 3 to 5 mornings per week. I lost about 15 or 20 pounds, and felt real good. I still ate whatever I wanted, and still was at least 50 pounds overweight. After paleo, I started doing pushups, pull-ups, deadlifts, walking, and sprinting. The problem is that I am very un-committed to a schedule. But even slacking for days in a row, it doesn't really seam to hurt my weight maintenance. I have lost a total of 85 pounds now, and I'm keeping it off. And I am eating all the real food my heart desires.

There were a lot people who doubted me in the beginning – who have now shut the hell up. You can't argue with real results. Most of them would say "you can't sustain this way of eating" and "eventually, you will go back to eating junk, and you'll gain it all back plus more." And of course the classic "you'll be dead within 6 months if you eat bacon and eggs every single day." Well, I'm still here, 2 years later, dipping my bacon in pure butter, and looking and feeling damn fine. And my physical transformation speaks for itself.

On the other side, there are also a lot of people who have gone paleo after seeing my success. Some have had great success, while others are still trying to break the bad habit of convenience. No one said it was a walk in the park. You do have to spend a lot more time in the kitchen cooking and cleaning. But hey, after a while, it just becomes "the way." And

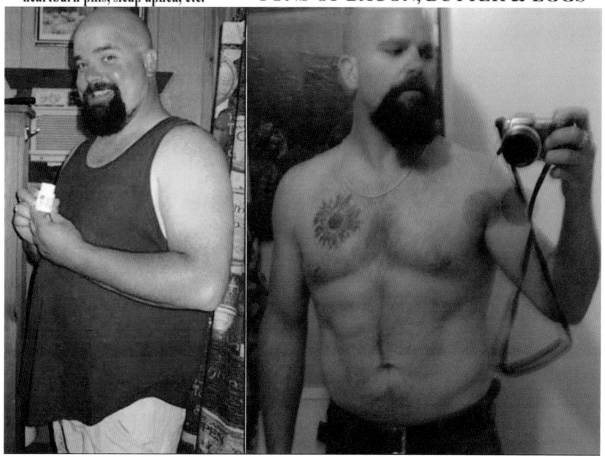

lots of healthy whole grains
standard american diet
heartburn pills, sleap apnea, etc.

18 months, no grains or sugars
exercise once every week or 2
TONS OF BACON, BUTTER & EGGS

boy, the food sure is good.

The last time I went to the general doc, it was about the very first month of going grain-free. I mentioned it to him, and he was not at all supportive. He wanted to take my blood, but I declined. I was about 80 pounds heavier that day then I am now. I ought to go pay him a visit…. but what the hell for? I am healthy inside and out.

MELISSA FRITCHER

SAN JOSE, CALIFORNIA

Before I went paleo, at 34 years old, I weighed in at a whopping 330 pounds and suffered from a plethora of debilitating health problems: I was a Type 2 Diabetic, with tests showing pancreatic function shutting down; I had high blood pressure for nearly 20 years; high cholesterol; arthritis; sleep apnea that led to near-narcoleptic episodes, and cost me my driver's license; gastro-intestinal problems ranging from acid reflux to IBS; hair loss (head, eyebrows, and eyelashes); emotional issues and hormonal imbalances including bipolar disorder and major depression; pre-menstrual dysphoric disorder (PMDD), and poly-cystic ovarian syndrome (PCOS). At the height of my ill health and obesity, I was on insulin, several medications and supplements for the diabetes (Metformin) and high blood pressure (Lisinopril), as well as three herbal supplements for mood stability. I could not exercise at the time because of the physical pain my excessive size caused, and my erratic blood sugar levels.

Before paleo, I was your typical obese person, eating for all the wrong reasons, at the wrong times, and doing absolutely no activity to combat the huge excess in refined carb, chemical, and caloric intake. It didn't help that I was labeled "disabled" after a back injury 15 years ago, because it gave me a very convenient excuse to be a couch-potato. My food intake at the time revolved around fast food restaurants, convenient pre-packaged foods, and tons of junk food, ice cream, candy, etc.

After the test results almost three years ago which showed my pancreas was losing functionality, I became extremely scared that I would eventually need to inject insulin just to live. I committed myself to a very low carb program, eating under 20 grams of carbohydrate a day, on a strict intake of just meat, eggs, and vegetables. I did very well on this for several months, but I was still reliant on my medications, and was still struggling with weight loss. A lot of my health problems - like the gastro-intestinal issues – continued to leave me feeling weak and malnourished.

I was very close to a paleo intake already, but there are some definite differences, mainly in that it's not all about the all-mighty "carb count" and paleo puts a larger emphasis on REAL food.

A friend suggested I try eliminating, for one month, the tiny portions of grains and sugars I had been eating just to see what would happen. I desperately wanted off the insulin and medications, and out of the obese category, so I decided to give it a shot. I cleaned up my eating using paleo guidelines and within a month, I was off insulin and all medications except the anti-depressants and the hypertension medications - and even those were reduced by half.

I eventually did get off all medications and supplements completely thanks to my paleo way of eating, and to date I've lost 99 pounds, with a goal of 60 more to go. I now make all my own meals and condiments - eat plenty of meat, eggs, vegetables, some fruit, some nuts, lots of good fats, including coconut oil, pastured butter, and bacon grease. I find I have better results if I focus on protein and vegetables only, but Paleo doesn't require counting or measuring food – so I don't.

The hardest part of changing my entire lifestyle to paleo has been mental. It took a very long time to accept that it is necessary for my health to be paleo for the rest of my life. I spent months dealing with all of my unhealthy psychological connections to foods that were detracting from my health. I had to learn new ways to deal with stress and emotional issues besides trying to eat them away. I felt amazing physically from very early on with these changes, but my mind has taken longer to catch up.

I'm now 37, I weigh 231, and my health is so much better. I recently went back on hypertension medication and anti-depressants because of a family loss, and I am confident that once the mourning period has passed that I will again be medication-free.

I no longer have any of the health issues I had before - my failing pancreas, diabetes, cholesterol, arthritis, sleep apnea, gastro-intestinal problems, hair loss, PMDD, and PCOS are

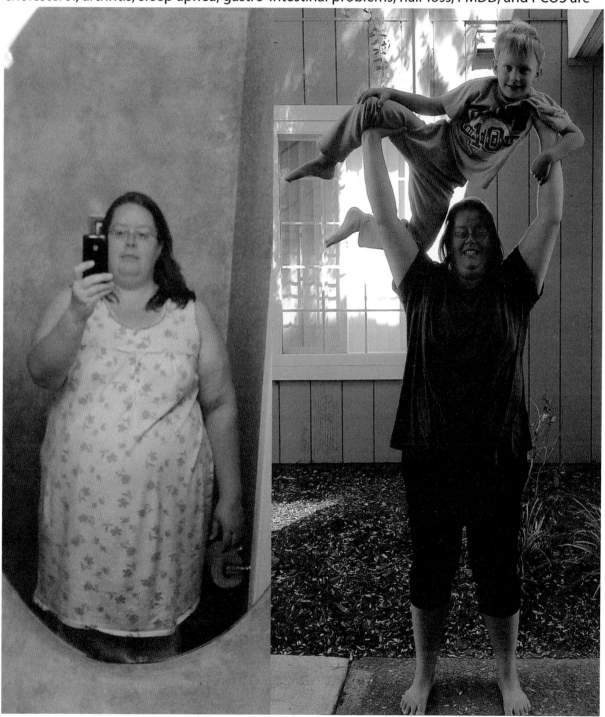

gone. I have also recently started exercising at a cross fit gym, at least three days a week, and have seen amazing improvements including enhanced back strength, and am well on the road to being perfectly healthy.

My family started out being quiet about my changes - likely because I'd done low-carb plans off and on for over 10 years with no real lasting success. When it became clear that this time was different and my health issues started disappearing, I got tons of support and praise. Several of my friends and family, including my husband and children, have all transitioned to paleo now, reaping their own rewards. Considering I got my life back, any challenges from people with respect to my diet are quickly quashed the moment I start discussing my progress.

I can say without hesitation eating paleo has saved my life, and it allows me to keep it on the best track.

The biggest difference is the combination of the physical, emotional, hormonal, and attitude changes that I have experienced the last two plus years. I feel alive for the first time in so long. I have a relationship with food that I treasure - I now believe that food should be viewed as fuel, preferably premium fuel that also tastes great. And, thanks to paleo, I know it also treats me well on the inside. I have more physical strength and ability than I have ever had. I am a better person overall - more balanced, vibrant, and happy. I am a better me, a better wife, mom, and friend. I love what paleo has done for me, and I show my love for it and my family by only providing them health-giving paleo foods.

I look back at how I felt at my un-healthiest, how I felt at my heaviest, and I know that I will never go back there. I have challenged and been victorious over so many personal issues in the last couple of years that I am empowered to explode through others that come my way. I'm a completely different person. I feel like I am finally who I was meant to be all my life. I have seized my life…and I'm going to run with it as far as I can.

ORLEATHA SMITH

LOS ANGELES, CALIFORNIA

www.lvlhealth.com

At 5', 4" my highest recorded weight, was 258 pounds. That was the weight taken at my annual physical with my general practitioner – who was at least 300 pounds himself. I wasn't sure how he could help me, but I felt that I had run out of options.

The problem was that I had been to Weight Watchers 6 (yes six) times. I had tried EVERY SINGLE DIET. *Seriously.* I was tired, and sick. I felt like bariatric surgery was my only option. I had to have a blood test in order to be considered and they confirmed what I had suspected – at 31 years old, I was borderline diabetic, had high blood pressure, high cholesterol, high triglycerides, and my stroke risk number was more than 5 times what it should have been.

I had to go through a series of meetings and consultations. I had what felt like a million pretests run. Finally, on 4/21/ 2009, I had my weight corrective surgery. Over the course of a year, I lost 90 pounds of my excess weight. I was steady at 165 pounds.

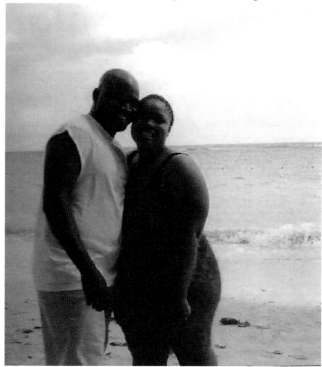

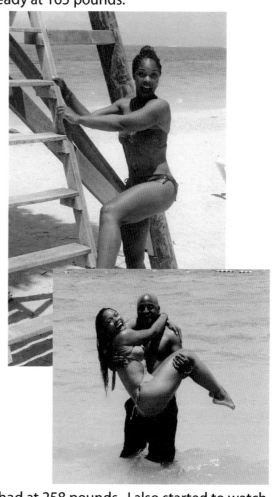

Jamaica
2004 (above)
2012 (at Right)

I knew I needed to lose more but I felt better than I had at 258 pounds. I also started to watch the scale start to creep back up. Instantly, I reverted back to my old diet mentality: I counted every calorie, gram of fat, ounce of carbs. I lost a pound, gained two; I lost two pounds, gained one back. It was maddening! Had I gone through ALL of that only to gain it back? Would I be banished to a life of low fat micro-meals, protein shakes, and calorie counting?? I ended up gaining almost 20 pounds back in my efforts to lose weight – again.

Enter this grain-free, sugar-free…this paleo lifestyle. The first week was hard. The second week was BLISS! I felt a burst of energy that I hadn't felt in what seemed like YEARS. At the end of the first month, I stepped on the scale and discovered that I had lost 15 pounds! WHAT??!? You mean I feel great AND lost weight? I had to stick to it!

Oh and I also reaped these benefits too:
My acute eczema has been under control WITHOUT the use of corticosteroids! The tendinitis in my Achilles has vanished! My asthma is gone! My once super-irregular cycle is like clock work – and not a cramp in sight!!! I wake up before the alarm clock daily – with energy to spare!

I am currently a size 2/4 and I have successfully lost over 125 pounds – and am keeping it off!

Check out my website Level Health and Nutrition at www.lvlhealth.com for delicious recipes and more!

TONY FEDERICO

FLORIDA

www.livecaveman.com

For the past year and a half, I have been happily living the paleo lifestyle. During this time, I have discovered the joys of coconut oil, explored organ meats, and "bulletproofed" my coffee. However, there hasn't been a significant change in my weight, body fat, cholesterol, or blood sugar. I can't say that paleo helped me to lose 100 pounds, cured my GERD, or transformed my physique into something akin to carved granite. To understand my paleo miracle, I need take you a little deeper, traveling back in time to where it all began:

Ten years ago, my life was in shambles. I was trapped in the cycle of addiction (toxic substances as well as and toxic relationships) and felt intensely uncomfortable any time sobriety or solitude forced me into self-reflection. The sense of control that I so desperately sought slipped further and further away and, as often happens, I hit my own personal rock bottom. The proverbial moment of clarity came by the realization that I could no longer manage my life on my own. Despite my pride, I accepted help and support from my family and slowly started to turn my life around.

It was during this time that I also experienced the unexpected and tragic death of a close friend. This was the first time I had experienced the death of someone who wasn't sick, self-destructive, or elderly. She was vital and effervescent. She loved life and had so much excitement for living it. It was devastating for her family and her friends. I cried for the first time in years. I cried until I felt completely wrung out and empty. I cried until there was nothing left but dry sobs and my face burned from wiping away tears.

I don't know if there is a purpose for events such as this, and feel like it would be selfish to say so. But, with her death and loss so raw and so close, I came to feel an even deeper responsibility to respect the gift that was my own life. At that time, I wouldn't have considered myself to be a good person. I cheated, lied, and manipulated with impunity, but I knew that love was there too. I loved my friend deeply and felt her love even after she was gone. This feeling gave me the strength to believe that maybe there was something good inside me after all.

Motivated by the desire to heal my own body, mind, and spirit, I pursued a degree in Exercise Science and graduated with honors. I also met the woman who is now my wife and who reminds me daily of how lucky I am to be alive. This was the start of my own personal transformation and launched my career in the fitness industry. It was a process of fits and

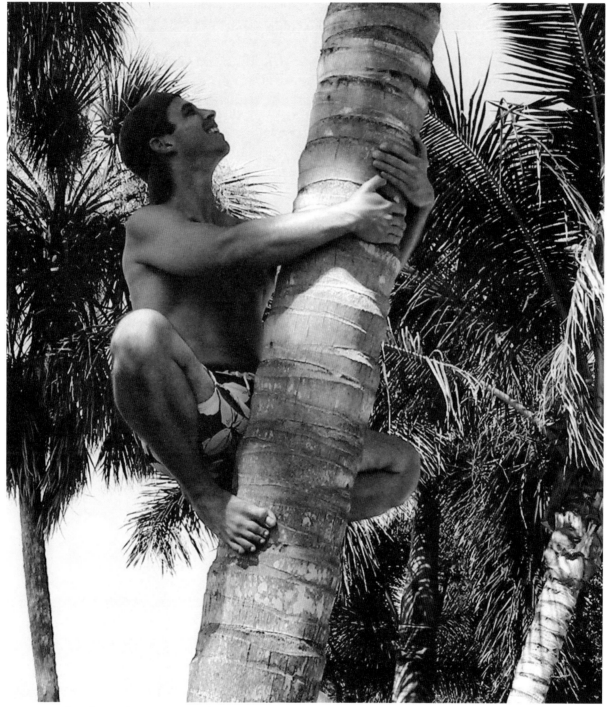

starts, setbacks and successes, disappointments and renewed determination, and just when I thought I had it "all figured out", a client of mine gave me a book called *The Paleo Diet*.

The notion there was "a universal human diet" was too compelling to ignore. I figured if zoo animals got sick and suffered ill health from eating unnatural foods, why wouldn't the same be true of humans? Eager to put this theory to the test, I embarked on my own personal 30-day paleo challenge. I was already eating a very nutrient-dense diet at the time, so the biggest change came by way of ditching my morning oatmeal and other whole grain products. Alcohol, chocolate, and dairy were also eliminated. This left a wide variety of fruits, veggies, nuts, eggs, and lean meats, all of which I ate without restriction.

The most immediate effect was a sense of dramatically increased energy and focus. As a teenager, I had been diagnosed as having ADD, and although I no longer took prescription drugs to treat it, it had continued to be a challenge. With paleo, however, my mind cleared dramatically, and I felt like it was easier to pay attention and accomplish tasks. As strange as it may seem, I also felt friendlier and more confident, as if the dial on my lingering social anxiety had been turned down. These changes prompted me to extend my experiment and the initial 30-day challenge turned into three months.

Towards the end of this 90 day experiment, however, I started to notice some undesirable effects. Specifically, I found that my sex drive had decreased significantly. This was disconcerting to say the least, but rather than give up completely, I decided to seek additional sources of information. Ultimately, I discovered Mark Sisson's *The Primal Blueprint* and Robb Wolf's *The Paleo Solution*. Both books stressed the importance of creating an optimal lifestyle, not just an optimal diet, so with a bit of trepidation, I cut back on my "chronic cardio," set a sleep timer (an alarm to remind me when to go to bed), started practicing Olympic lifts, and beefed up my fat intake. Literally, I started eating lots of fatty beef - and it felt great! My sex drive returned, my strength increased, and I found that the dark circles that had ringed my eyes like a raccoon for years began to disappear.

Encouraged by this progress, I decided to go even deeper in my studies of what it means to live "primally." I conducted numerous self-experiments and read a great many books on Evolutionary Biology, Evolutionary Psychology, Ecology, and Anthropology. I began to look at the entire world through a different lens and realized that eating a Paleo diet was only the beginning of my journey. I realized how fundamental the experiences of tribe, nature, storytelling, music, and even fire were to humankind and sought these types of authentic experiences in my own life.

On another level, I began to reflect upon my own personal struggles in a new light. I had always tried to be "in control", to use the sheer force of my will to "make" the world fit my expectations. This inevitably backfired, but with my new evolutionary perspective, I realized that by setting the right environment, one that surrounded my body with the foods and experiences that it was designed to thrive in, I could let go of control without going out of control. I could eat a meal and feel satiated. I could take a day off of working out without feeling guilty for having failed to "burn calories". I could take a walk with nothing between my feet and the ground, I could feel the sun on my bare skin, I remembered what it was like to play.

This is my personal Paleo Miracle, and although I don't look much different than I did before, on the inside, I'm a completely different animal.

LEIGH GARCIA

PHILADELPHIA, PENNSYLVANIA

paleoatpenn.blogspot.com

I struggled with my weight up until the age of 18. I was a chubby kid – I was a women's size 8/10 in fourth grade, and a size 18 by the seventh grade. Starting in January of 2004, I spent six months doing the Atkins Diet for the first time, and lost about thirty pounds. Like many dieters, however, I gained it all back, plus a lot more.

When I went to high school, I stopped dancing ballet twice a week, started working at Dunkin' Donuts, and by the summer before my junior year, I was 200 pounds and a size 18 again. I did the Atkins Diet once again for a few months and spent the next two years around a size 14. I was always tired, became ravenously hungry just a few hours after every meal, had bad acne, and spent most of every winter with a cold. Despite the fact I was overweight, I thought I was in relatively good health because I never had any major health problems.

The summer before my freshman year of college I did Atkins again and dropped some more weight—I moved into my dorm wearing a size 12. Like most college kids, I went crazy in the dining hall and put on the "freshman fifteen." Although I was more active and walked everywhere, I was so out of shape that I could never make it up the twelve flights of stairs to my dorm. I always took the elevator.

On January 31, 2010, just after my nineteenth birthday, I was feeling sluggish and gross from eating a ton of food over the holidays. I had spent the first few weeks of the new semester pigging out in the dining hall as usual. This night was particularly memorable because I remember that for dinner I ate a bowl of Fruity Pebbles, and was starving an hour later. I went out to a local sandwich place called Wawa and bought a hoagie. After finishing it, I felt even more disgusting and knew that this absolutely needed to stop. I decided to go on Atkins again and said to myself, "Tomorrow is going to be the first day of the rest of my life."

The next day, February 1, 2010, actually turned out to be the first day of the rest of my life. I traded in my bowl of cereal every morning for scrambled eggs. I went from eating pizza or sandwiches for lunch to salads or non-breaded protein dishes. I went from pasta (or cereal) for dinner to bun-less burgers. I called what I was doing Atkins, but it was really paleo – I only ate animal protein, veggies, and healthy fats.

I stayed very, very strict on this new diet. After a month and a half, I had lost about twenty pounds and was a size 8/10, and I knew that I couldn't look back now—I would never wind up 200 pounds again! I started moving more – to the point where not only could I climb the twelve flights of stairs to my floor, but I could climb all twenty-four in my building! – and unknowingly started intermittent fasting by stopping breakfast, only eating lunch and dinner to fit my hunger level.

By the end of the semester, I had gone down to a size 6 and had lost about 50 pounds! I had so much more energy, my acne completely went away, and I didn't get sick at all that last half of winter or in the spring! I was back to wearing my "skinny clothes" from that first post-Atkins attempt in seventh grade!

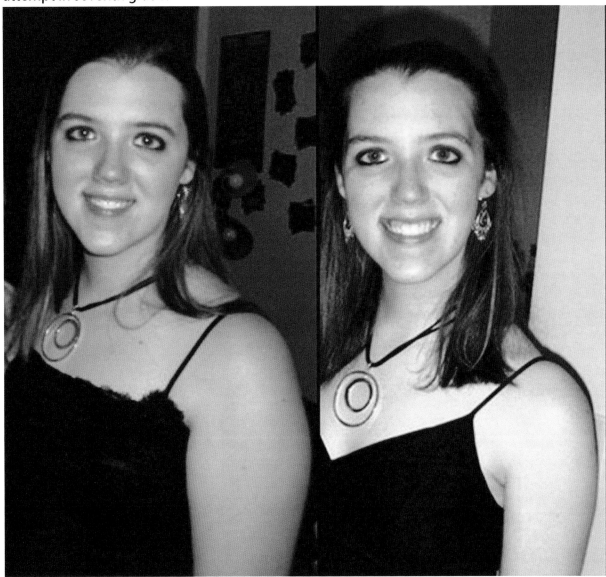

Eating paleo also encouraged me to try new foods. Up until that point in my life, I was a very picky eater and wouldn't eat most vegetables. But because I was really only eating animal protein and lettuce, I decided to try some new vegetables, and absolutely fell in love with them! I discovered how delicious tomatoes and onions and mushrooms are. I got hooked on broccoli and cauliflower. Although there are still some foods I won't eat (such as fish), I'm a much more adventurous eater now!

Eating just animal protein and veggies in a college setting was really difficult—I no longer went out for ice cream with my friends, temptation was around every corner (almost every college event has pizza, soda, and/or sugary snacks), and I felt very alone and isolated because I refused to put myself into situations where I might slip up. My friends thought I was insane, and I got the "Oh, c'mon, you can just have one bite!" line a million times, but I never gave in. I was—and still am—a sugar addict, and "just one bite" would get me up to 200 pounds again. For the first time ever, I put my health above everything else.

My family was incredibly supportive—my dad has been eating Weston Price-style since the mid-90s, so with the two of us eating so healthily all the time, my mom got on board and lost a ton of weight as well. Today, we only have paleo meals in my house!

I didn't really discover what "paleo" was until January 2011 when my dad read Loren Cordain's *The Paleo Diet* and sent me a copy with a "This is how you eat!" note attached. From there, I read all of the other paleo literature available at the time (by Robb Wolf, Art DeVany, and Mark Sisson), and learned the science behind the food I was (and was not) eating, as well as the benefits of grass-fed meat and eating locally. I was so shocked that there was an entire movement centered on the way I eat, and was so excited that I jumped right in after reading other blogs and started my own blog, Paleo at Penn (paleoatpenn.blogspot.com) which discusses this lifestyle and my experiences as a college student.

It has been over two and a half years since I began my journey to health, and I'm never going back to my old lifestyle. I haven't gotten sick since February 2010, I rarely have acne, I can go many hours without eating, I have a ton of energy, and I just feel really healthy. I now walk a lot more and lift weights a few times a week, have enough control to go out with my friends and say no to sugary foods, and probably know more about nutrition than most doctors. Although this journey started out as another diet, it has been—and always will be—a lifestyle.

SARA GUSTAFSON EYE

BUDA, TEXAS

sara.eye@gmail.com

My name is Sara, and I grew up in Austin, Texas. I am 32 years old and currently weight about 118 pounds, which tends to fluctuate quite often. However, I no longer step on the scale - so I usually gauge my weight by the size of my jeans.

Back in 1987, I was a shaky, sick, and miserable seven-year-old kid living in Fredericksburg, Virginia. The youngest of four, I was often the target of intolerance from my siblings due to my behavior problems and chronic illnesses. Medical interventions finally stopped working when I became resistant to all antibiotics and landed in the hospital for several weeks - all because of an ear infection. Because I was resistant to antibiotics at such a young age, even adult dosages, the infection began to spread to my brain. I felt much better after I was admitted, hooked up to some machines, and had round-the clock care.

After leaving the hospital, my life resumed, but it was the beginning of a long and rocky childhood (if you can call it that). By age 10 I had my first migraine. A full-on legit migraine. I remember the day exactly because I was in fourth grade and became confused when I suddenly could not see out of my right eye. I asked my teacher Mrs. Bean to help me walk to the nurse. I was scared I was going blind. I laid down and waited for my mom to pick me up and by then the blindness had turned into a crazy, flashing light show and when I tried to open my eyes, the light seemed to stab me straight into the eyeball.

That same year I was plagued with insomnia. Imagine an eighty-pound, ten-year-old kid moving a box spring and mattress, on her own, into her closet in order to create two walls between her and her older sister who talked on the phone all hours of the night. This didn't even work, because even the sound of my own breathing kept me awake. I cried for hours in frustration so many nights, and as a result, my family thought I was crazy. None of them could understand that the smell of smoke, or the sound of murmuring through the walls could literally ignite a migraine, which I was often accused of faking, or that it could literally keep me wide awake all night long driving me into crazed fits. No one got it.

This is how I entered my pre-teens, where hormones just made my conditions worse. I missed so much school between seventh grade and junior year in high school because of migraines, insomnia, depression, anxiety, and infections that seemed to heal but always returned in four to six weeks. It was like clockwork. Every time I finished a round of antibiotics you could literally guess the date and time when the infection would return. By age fifteen, I was being pumped with steroids. This caused an awkward weight gain and massive skin lesions and acne. I never wanted to leave the house. I was no longer the fastest runner on the soccer team and was demoted from mid-field to stopper. It was a crushing blow to my ego, and because I never could seem to catch up with health and compete shoulder-to-shoulder with my peers, my self-confidence took a nosedive - which led to poor grades and poor performance.

By age 17 I was on anti-depressants. By then, the doctors had no other explanation to my chronic health problems other than "it's all in her head" and started me on Prozac. That year was just a fog and I don't remember much of it. Once I moved away to college, I stopped taking all my medications and ended up feeling a lot better. However, recurring injuries to the joints and ligaments ended my dreams of playing soccer again.

In the first two years of college, I had switched majors three times, dropped and added classes countless times, and secluded myself to a small apartment closed off from most of the world. I had no confidence in my future whatsoever. I had missed the boat on being properly diagnosed with ADHD and was allowing that to spiral out of control. The only way I found control in my life was to maintain 2-3 jobs at a time (seriously) while attending school. This never gave me much bandwidth to perform my best, but if left too much free time I would spiral even worse.

By 2001, my third year in college, I had become incredibly sick and unable to recover, and ended up returning home to Austin where I attended a university near my parent's home. Within a year I had dropped down to 101 pound, my hair was falling out, and the migraines increased to 4 times a week. Insomnia owned me, anxiety was all time high, I was bloated, in pain, depressed, tired, moody, and incapable of concentrating. I finally saw a specialist who performed an endoscopy, and he told me that although celiac disease is rare, I had one of the worst cases he had ever seen. He had to remove a benign tumor from my esophagus and gave me radiation treatments as a precautionary control and sent me on my way only explaining "don't eat gluten". And when I asked him what gluten was he said "Google it". That was it. That was my diagnosis and instruction.

Four years later, I was living and working in Washington, DC on Capitol Hill, working various low-paying jobs trying to get my foot in the congressional door. In 2004 I was diagnosed with Fibromyalgia. Out of frustration, I began doing my own research at that point on diet and nutrition. I discovered the SCD diet, which is similar to the paleo diet, only more strict. This was the ONLY time to date I had ever felt better in my life. I often ate on-the-go from cafes downtown, which consisted of hard boiled eggs, oatmeal, yogurt or fruit. I drank a lot of coffee! In an effort to stick to a specific-carbohydrate plan, I switched from eating out at restaurants with my husband four times a week and shoveling as many concoctions of cardboard-tasting gluten free breads and snacks into my mouth to suddenly buying foods that expired much sooner. I went from longer shelf-life pantry items and packaged flour mixes to things I had to keep in the refrigerator and eat within 3-5 days. If I had not eaten this way prior to discovering paleo, it definitely would have taken me longer to adjust. I learned that it takes BABY STEPS to transition your life from a very pre-packaged and on-the-go lifestyle to a healthy one, and labels associated with a way of eating are secondary.

Before eating paleo, I weighed about 118 pounds and wore a size four. Five years later, I still weigh 118 pounds, but wear a size two! I was painfully thin prior to embracing the paleo lifestyle and jiggly with a poor complexion and zero energy. The fact that my weight has remained the same but my jean size has gone down demonstrates how malnourished I was before. I never had enough nutrition (or the ability to absorb) to even form muscle.

Paleo has changed my life in so many ways that a year ago I decided to change my career path. I was aggressively pursuing a juvenile probation officer position in the criminal justice system and instead become certified in Sports Conditioning and Training as well as Holistic Nutrition.

Once I was able to heal myself by eating paleo, I was awakened to the very simple, yet so crucial, point: Everything starts with food. Not only did I come off six medications for insomnia, migraines, pain, depression, and anxiety (which saves me a total of $216 a month), but I could now also see clearly that food was destroying the health of my most beloved family members.

In 2010, my father was on his 3rd heart stent, my mother was diagnosed with Type II Diabetes, my youngest daughter and I both got the Swine Flu (despite both having the vaccinations), and by age 2 she was also diagnosed with celiac disease. Right around the same time my dearest and closest Aunt, who was like a second mother to me, was diagnosed with stage IV colon cancer. As I watched my Aunt slowly, and painfully die from this disease I realized my passion about life had changed. Suddenly I went from thinking (and accepting) that I'll probably die around the age of 75 and likely from some form of cancer to understanding that my choices could honestly prolong my life long enough to watch my great grandchildren graduate college. And that became my new reality. No, I DO NOT have to die or get cancer.

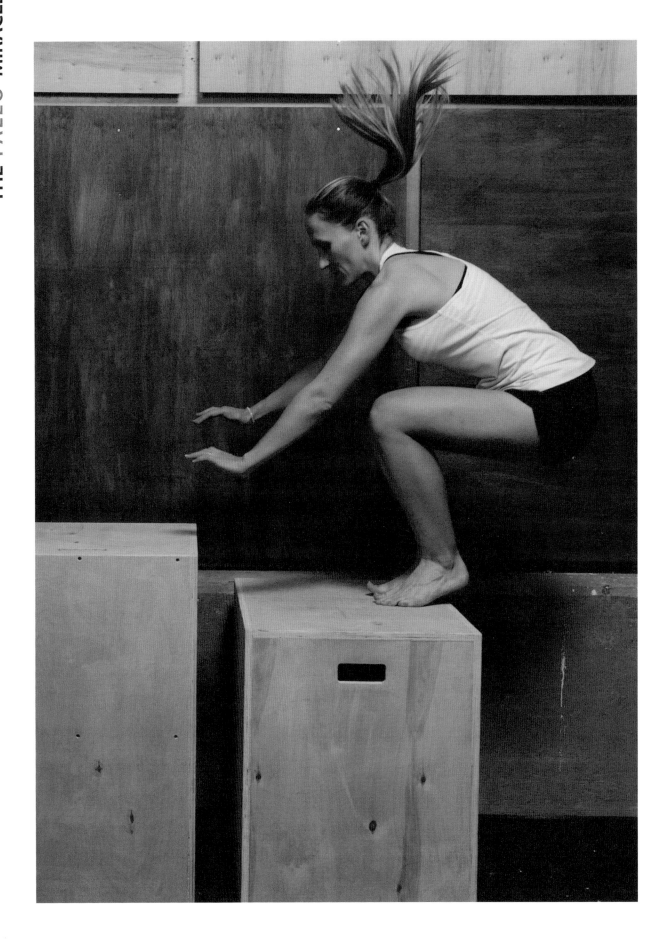

Neither does my family.

A year after eating a paleo protocol, I have been able to convince my mother to switch into this lifestyle. And though it has taken over 6 months, I have transitioned my two daughters to eating an 80/20 paleo plan. The results: my oldest daughter now sleeps through the night and is able to concentrate in school. It has dramatically improved her behavior as well. The youngest is not dealing with so many illnesses as she did the first 2 years of her life, and in fact you could label her "healthy" now, thank God. My mother, who was on ELEVEN prescription medications, has already eliminated three of them and is slowly coming off all of the rest, one at a time. My father has adopted the "paleo mindset" but has not given up sugar completely... but being a man, he was able to lose 3 inches in just 2 weeks by simply cutting out gluten and corn.

The most important thing to me in all of this has been the ability to live a NORMAL life without the fear and reservation associated with getting migraines on a daily basis, or waking up in severe pain because I did not sleep the night before. I can make plans and be confident I can perform, attend, and follow through on them without having to call and explain another health issue.

MARTY WILSON

CHANDLER, ARIZONA

mw@martywilson.us

There were hints; there were truths hidden along with untruths; there was a glimmer of what a paleo lifestyle held in store for me prior to that day about exactly two years ago that I was introduced to paleo. Due to studies in nutrition, cultural and physical anthropology, I had an idea that something was out there, but it was hidden under contradictory theories. I was also somewhat involved in the Caloric Restriction movement and considered myself quite knowledgeable.

I, however, was not. And my body showed evidence of it – big time. After over four years of the deleterious effects of a fairly decent foray into vegetarianism (including a number of years as a vegan), my body was not what it used to be. I gained forty pounds and suffered from acute systemic inflammation. I also eventually either became celiac or simply had an extreme chronic allergic reaction to gluten. I have been gluten-free for over 2.5 years and all of the extreme ills that I suffered while eating gluten have disappeared.

To name a few: I had five or six episodes of anaphylaxic shock with my throat closing up almost completely. I also had six or seven episodes of extreme stomach cramps (somewhat common celiac symptoms). I was unable to move and curled up in a fetal position for hours. It wasn't until I found that antihistamine relieved the symptoms that I received relief much more quickly. I had some type of auto-immune response to my 'healthy' SAD diet. At one point, I also had an extreme case of 'weeping sores' on my right arm that made it impossible to bend at the elbow for weeks. I also experienced intermittent hives on various parts of my body.

Also, a few years before finding paleo, I had many months of extreme inflammation in my right arm. I was unable to type at the computer without extreme pain; I could not play the piano, and I could not sing due to inflammation in my throat. I was a mess and I thought my life was pretty much over. And it is no exaggeration that it very nearly ended due to the anaphylaxic shock. I also suffered from tinnitus (which is especially horrible) and chronic sleep apnea. I also had episodes of severe back-pain that debilitated me for hours and caused pain for days.

Additionally, there were bouts of brain-fog and emotional outbursts due to the inflamed state of my body, including my brain. Stress was, at times, excruciatingly unbearable and as a primary care-giver for my invalid mother for over six years, and being employed full-time as an executive, I needed all the fortitude I could muster. It is also no exaggeration that life itself was becoming virtually unbearable.

As of today, September of 2012, at 57 years old, I am 90% Paleo with a 'work-in-progress' elimination of sugary sweets. I have lost thirty-three pounds. I am unusually energetic and physically strong for my age (I can do squats, whereas before – as with most middle-aged women – I avoided them). I am more athletic and toned, more clear thinking, happier, more productive, and more radiant. I have more time for my family obligations and I cook more. I am more focused on high-quality meats & fish (like jerky, dried salmon, and organ meats); steamed, grilled or fresh vegetables (mostly sweet potatoes, squash, onion, peppers, garlic, kale, spinach); free-range non-vegetarian eggs; coconut products; fermented foods; oils (avoiding industrialized seed oils); infrequent high-quality cheese; occasional baked non-grain Paleo treats; dark chocolate; high quality butter and Himalayan sea salt. I also sometimes still eat candy, which I am working on eliminating from my diet. At this point, thankfully, it has not caused any weight-gain.

What is most exciting is how my activities and employment have changed. I now, thanks completely to paleo, am able to sing and play the piano again. I teach close to full-time and have found that health issues (particularly allergies) are very important to monitor for a musical career. I also assist a small number of people with a paleo lifestyle and am working on creating a paleo immersion program. My day is full of work that I want to do – rather than work that only brings in a paycheck. I also am more active in nature; have a bigger garden than previously and have more time for my artistic endeavors.

Surprisingly, when I am strict paleo, I can *see* clearer. This makes life a lot easier. My activities are enhanced by my newly-discovered ability to see unaided by glasses. I only use very mild reading glasses when I am eating more sugar than usual.

Amazingly, any hint of tinnitus is very mild and infrequent (if I do get it, it's clearly traceable to consuming sugary snacks). This *one thing by itself makes it worthwhile*. I guess it's not the worst thing that can befall a person – but ringing in your ears that you cannot escape is really horrible. Finally, my teeth are so much stronger, and I have escaped excess difficulties with dental caries. My gums have become far less inflamed thanks to paleo.

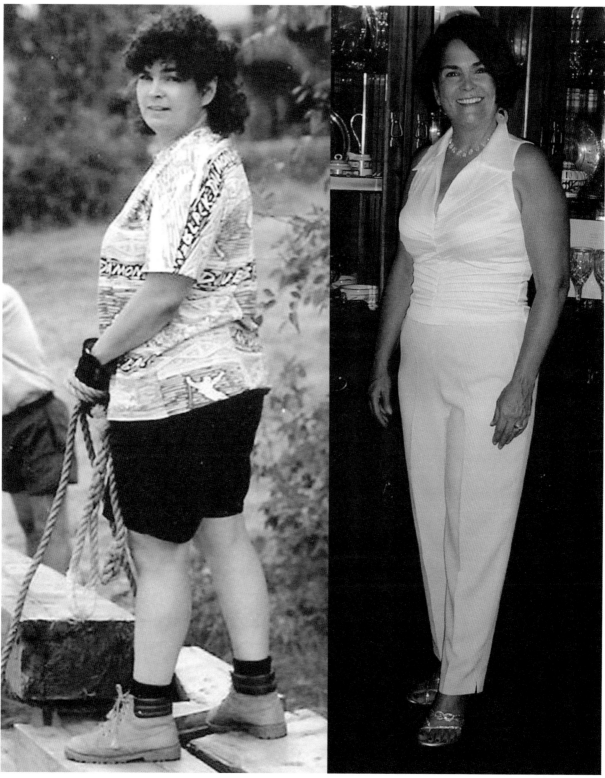

As far as I am concerned, Paleo has been a true life-saver and life-enhancer for me. I now feel that I can make good on my promise of living to 120 as a vibrant, happy, mentally-clear, disease-free woman. Words cannot express my gratitude for this lifestyle. It makes it possible for the legacy of my life to reach a higher potential than without it.

MISTY HUMPHREY

SONOMA COUNTY, CALIFORNIA

www.healthy-transitions.com , freehealthydietplans@gmail.com

I often wonder what my life would be like had I not finally turned my dieting *career* into a healthy lifestyle. A lower carbohydrate paleo diet has literally saved my life. I am now 48 years old and weigh 130 pounds.

By the time I was 14 years old, I had undergone two exploratory surgeries. The first surgery revealed an ovarian cyst and the second, from what I can determine now, gastritis. The physician removed my appendix "for good measure", sewed me back up and my Mother insinuated that I was faking my symptoms. The problem was that I was chronically constipated, suffered gastric distress, and developed a Tourette style tic along with ADHD & OCD behaviors

This was the early 1970s – and information was limited both medically as well as psychologically. In retrospect, I'm thankful. Other than several rounds of antibiotics for various strep infections and hormone therapy for the PCOS, no other medications were offered to me. Today's children going through the same thing would likely be offered a handful of drugs. I now understand that my diet and my behavior were and are directly linked.

I was about 15-20 pounds overweight for most of my childhood. My Mother was conscious not only about her weight, but mine as well. We went on diets frequently but they were always fad diets to lose weight – only to discontinue it after several weeks or upon arrival of an event we had been dieting for. My best memory of dieting was the TWA Stewardess diet that was quite popular in the 1970s. What do I remember most? That I was always hungry. I remember constantly thinking about food. A box of candy, a plate of fudge or cookies, I would try to eat as much as I could as frequently as possible. If any food was in the room, it was constantly on my mind.

As a child, I remember fainting a couple of times. Other times I felt out of control – all the while constantly hungry and, consequently, irritable. I had no idea that I was having blood sugar balance issues until I began studying nutrition.

Fast forward several years, many diets later, and I was still un-focused and a smoker, consuming too much alcohol, and 215 pounds on my 5' 4" frame. It was time once again for Weight Watchers. I was successful with this diet after my third child – but never without the assistance of diet pills. I had what I thought was a ravenous appetite all the time – but made it partially work anyway through guilt. Each diet I chose was notoriously a low fat diet and I had major cravings and constant hunger of which I could not function on.

Follow-through and perseverance are not virtues of the typical ADHD person unless there is a great deal of interest. Moreover, the ADHD person is also more inclined to become addicted to substances such as appetite suppressants and most particularly "uppers" – like diet pills.

Yes, I was that statistic. We all have our dirty little secrets to try to achieve goals – and hopefully if I share mine, you will realize that there is an easier, more efficient way.

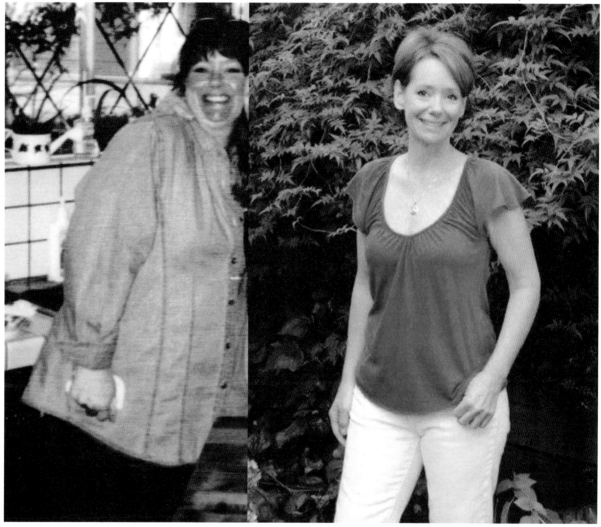

My husband and I always shopped together and tried to make healthy choices – usually serving chicken and vegetables – but it was always low-fat or non-fat with plenty of bread. Like most parents, we did the best we could with the information we had. These were the years I followed the USDA food pyramid and low fat diet advice. I even tried a vegan diet for a stint.

I finally figured out that whole wheat sandwich rolls and loads of vegetables didn't feed me efficiently despite the fact that my doctor was convinced that this was the right diet for humans.

On February 7th of 2000, I started the Atkins Diet. In the first few days of increasing my animal proteins and fats, and eating 2-3 cups of vegetables daily, I was a new person. The weight began falling off, my energy levels soared, my focus became clear, and I was not hungry! Never had I felt like this on any other diet in my life.

I eventually learned that I was practicing paleo, and the more I learned the more confident I was that I could maintain a paleo lifestyle.

Thanks to the work of many (especially Robb Wolf for the plethora of information he gives to the community) I figured out that my digestive disorder began from not breast feeding, then from being given baby formula, and that it was perpetuated by gluten. The tic I had was a result of gluten intolerance, and I am excited to report that the tic is gone.

During my transition, my husband not only witnessed my transformation but very patiently listened to me while I regurgitated the information I was learning. He is a smart man, and that made it easy for him to make the transition with me.

We are a very happy paleo couple, completely free of prescription drugs, using natural foods and body movement as our medicine.

ADAM FARRAH

OLD SAYBROOK, CONNECTICUT

http://is.gd/missinglink

In the fall of 2004 I owned a big house with a big mortgage, worked a high-stress corporate biotech job, slept fewer than 5-6 hours a night and had just started an evening MBA program. I drank tons of coffee. Everything about my life was rushed and stressed. Of course, everyone would have expected me to remain healthy despite the schedule and the stress – after all, I was working out all the time, jogging almost daily and eating a "very healthy" diet of chicken breasts, protein shakes, whole grains, protein bars, granola bars, name brand yogurt and taking plenty of vitamins and supplements.

Next thing I know, I almost died from Ulcerative Colitis, and I began a long battle with digestive illness, chronic fatigue, depression and a lot of other health issues. Of course I, and anyone in the mainstream establishment I knew, attributed my problems to "bad luck." All the doctors I saw except one couldn't – and wouldn't – do anything to help me except medicate my symptoms with drugs that usually made things worse or caused other problems. I was told over and over again: "There's no known cause for your illness and no known cure. All we can do is 'manage your disease' with drugs. Diet has nothing to do with it." I even had the head of Gastroenterology at a major university hospital recommend I eat "bread" because my diet of only raw fruit smoothies and steamed vegetables – which seemed to be making me feel better and reduce the pain of digestion – wasn't of adequate nutrition and nutrient "deficiencies" might result without bread.

I also made the rounds to various alternative medicine practitioners. All of them proved useless and were only interested in selling high-priced supplements or advancing their own dogmatic ideas. None had any answers, but all were more than happy to accept money in exchange for a useless opinion, some tests, and some useless bottles of crap that didn't help and sometimes made me feel worse.

I spent YEARS of my life sick and exhausted. My usually boundless creativity and energy were gone. I could barely drag myself to a job that I hated so I could sit at a desk and collect a paycheck. I still worked out and did Karate, but my training was lackluster and always interrupted for various time periods by digestive problems from moderate to severe. I made more than one trip to an emergency room due to dehydration, anemia and severe inflammation of my intestinal tract. Each time it was the same story: "Diet has nothing to do with it. You'll need to be on medication for the rest of your life to 'manage your disease.'"

My grandfather once said about me: "Adam is over-confident and over-optimistic, but he usually turns out to be right." Looking back it was pretty crazy – I stopped taking the prednisone and other crap they were loading me up with, stopped looking to others for help, and began reading everything I could get my hands on and experimenting. I experimented with all sorts of diets, fasting, positive thinking, meditation and everything else that had even a remote chance of helping me. Every so often, I'd show up in an emergency room because things got out of hand. I'd do just enough conventional treatment to get back on my feet and get back to my still-stressful job and resume my dietary research and trial and error.

This was all nearly 7 years ago. It's relatively easy to talk about now, but the day to day process I went through was excruciating. Over that 7 years I examined every aspect of my diet, my past, my goals, my thinking, my friends, my relationships, my work and my life. It was a battle and I was literally fighting for my life. And not just my "life" as in not dying, my life as in having a good one that I enjoyed and actually wanted to live. I have no doubt that the doctors could have kept me alive – but I'm certain the life I would have had under their care would have been a living hell.

I eventually reached the point where I was determined to regain my health and live the life I wanted or die trying. There would be no lifetime of drugs and surgeries and emergency rooms and gastroenterologists who could barely speak English. They all told me I would die if I didn't take their medications and do what they told me. They told me that nothing I did with my diet or lifestyle would help. It was a risk I was willing to take. Life on my terms or death, those were my options. At times, I really didn't care which one it was.

Things began to really turn around in 2008, even though I was working yet another stressful and miserable corporate job and still had plenty of negative people and situations in my life. I was doing relatively well on a diet of meats, fruit, vegetables and goat yogurt and had been eating that diet for years. I was still far from healthy, though. At this time, I still thought my training days were over. I was too tired and too out of shape to want to do much of anything. I used to be big and strong and fit and live in the gym. College, then corporate life and then illness changed all that. I had lost all of the muscle and strength I built from a lifetime of weights and training. And now, the diet I needed to be on to stay healthy wasn't anything like the one I "needed" to be on to get strong and train again. Or so I thought.

Like most, I was deluded by marketing and mainstream nonsense. I thought there was a specific diet you ate for each health problem, a diet you ate to build muscle, a diet you ate to burn fat, a diet you ate for psychological health, a diet you ate to run marathons and on and on. Special diets and special supplements. Like everything else in our modern world, everything was specialized and fractionated as far as I could tell. Eating to heal a digestive illness may have been my priority at one time, but it was entirely ignorant of me – and of our culture in general – to think that the diet that healed my digestive system wouldn't be the diet that would help me achieve strength and performance or psychological health or any other goal I had. Certainly the application of certain principles or foods might change, but a healthy diet is a healthy diet regardless of goals or specific circumstances.

A healthy diet is a healthy diet and is universal. Let me say that again in a different way: *There are solid, unchanging principles that make up a diet that is healthy for humans. This is a fact. There is a right and a wrong way to eat.* Yes, there is latitude within the context of "what is a healthy diet to eat" and there will be differences and variations depending on goals, individual health, tolerance for certain foods, genetics and a million other details, but the question of what to eat is not as complex as many would like us to believe. In fact, science tells us – with absolute certainty – what is healthy for us to eat and what is not healthy for us to eat. It's just that the science that tells us this, sadly, isn't medical science. The science that gives us the answers to the questions we ask about what to eat is anthropology and the related disciplines. To see our way to a healthy future we need to use science to look at the past.

The idea of this diet vs. that diet, the 1000's of diet books, the experts and doctors and pundits and arguments and conflicts on TV and most everything else within the commercial diet landscape are nothing but distracting nonsense, bullshit, hype, and manipulative marketing efforts.

Evolution tells us how to eat and how to live. History shows us what we were designed to eat and how we were designed to live, and history shows us how we've declined as a species the further we've drifted from what is natural to us. Evolution shows us that we thrived for over 100,000 years when we were eating a specific diet.

"All truth passes through three stages. First, it is ridiculed. Second, it is violently opposed. Third, it is accepted as being self-evident." ~ Arthur Schopenhauer

Everything changed for me in 2009 when I read Randy Roach's book *Muscle, Smoke and Mirrors. Volume I.* In this outstanding history of bodybuilding and Physical Culture, Randy showed the diets and nutritional philosophies of the strongest and healthiest from the 1800's and early to mid 1900's, before modern medicine was what it is now, before marketing and medicating symptoms were what they are now. For the first time, I was aware of athletes who were capable of moving weights I couldn't have dreamed of in my best training days – and they were doing it long before anabolic steroids, "advanced" protein shakes and bars, pre-workout drinks and stimulants and all the equipment "advances" we are told we need to be strong and be healthy. Many of these men drank raw cow or goat milk, ate foods straight from the farms they were grown or raised on and practiced a lot of the "strange" things I read about in many of the very fringe books I was reading about health and healing. Many of them fasted, they obsessed about food quality. Many avoided grains. Most avoided alcohol. This is the first time I really saw the connection between eating for health and eating for strength and performance.

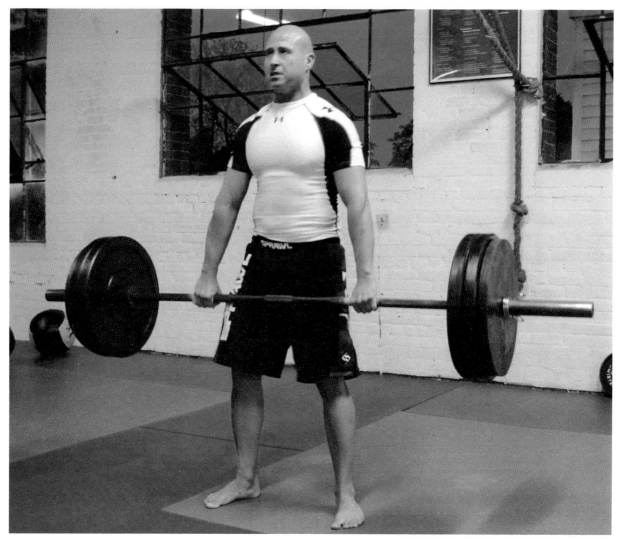

I also saw the connection between lifestyle and health or the lack of it. Once I started making these connections, things started to really pick up momentum and change in my life. I quit jobs and ended relationships. My friend Chris Wright-Martell let me start training clients as a strength coach out of his school, Modern Self-Defense Center in Middletown, CT. He had a few kettlebells at the school and I started using them. I got hooked. A few months later I got certified as Kettlebell Teacher by Steve Cotter and Ken Blackburn from the IKFF. I started training harder and feeling better.

It wasn't too long after this that I found my way to the CrossFit community when I taught a kettlebell seminar at CrossFit Relentless. I became good friends with the owner, Merle Mckenzie, and he encouraged me to get into CrossFit. I did. And that's when I came full circle. CrossFitters were eating Paleo and doing it for performance. I started following Robb Wolf's work.

In 2005 all my friends and coworkers wanted to know when I would be able to eat "normally" again. Girlfriends were annoyed and frustrated because there was "something wrong with me" that kept us from taking day trips to Sturbridge Village to eat fried seafood and ice cream.

They wanted to stay out all night and drink in loud clubs and I wanted to be home sleeping at 10pm – because there was "something wrong with me."

Today, I'm healthy. I'm happy. I live in the tiny beach cottage in Old Saybrook, CT that my great grandfather bought for the family as a summer home. I run at the beach. I feel good. I eat good local foods. I do yoga in the yard in the sun with humming birds flitting here and there. I go to bed early, I get up early and I lift heavy things in a little barn behind the house. I write constantly. I have a wonderful, spiritual woman in my life. I actively avoid negative people and places and practices. There's nothing "wrong with me" anymore. In truth, there never was anything "wrong with me." There was – and still is – something wrong with a culture where true health isn't a priority, foods we're told are healthy by "experts" aren't, disease is rampant, lifestyles are out of control with stress and strife and no one will look at the facts, tell the truth, drop the politics and create change. Misinformation in the diet and health fields is ubiquitous. Almost no one tells the truth. Almost.

The Paleo Dieter's Missing Link is my contribution to creating change in the way we think about health and diet and the way we eat and live. Some of the things I say in the book are risky and unpopular. It's a Paleo diet book but, as I'll show you, Paleo is a diverse diet genre. It's not a single diet made up of black and white principles to follow without question or individualization. I'm not here to make friends. I'm here to help you understand Paleo and related approaches in a way that they're not typically presented or explained. I want to empower you to make your own decisions, ask your own questions and find your own answers. I want to make connections and integrate knowledge from different places and different historical periods. I want to help you understand health and diet on a much deeper level than it's currently presented.

I had to understand diet, health and lifestyle to heal and live again. I understand it on a very deep level because of the stakes I was playing at. I had to because I couldn't have turned that mess of a life I was living around any other way. Many people still don't get me or my lifestyle or my diet, but that's really OK. I don't care. I'm living my life the way I want to live it and that's what's important. I'm living life on my terms…and I am healthier and happier for it.

CALE SCHULTZ

REDONDO BEACH, CALIFORNIA

caleschultz@gmail.com

For the last 15 years or so, I've been following the bodybuilder lifestyle to the best of my abilities. I've never competed, I just really enjoyed it. For me, that consisted of lifting weights, reading bodybuilding magazines, taking supplements, and eating protein. You live and you learn, and I have learned a lot, mostly through self-experimentation and trial and error. If only I knew then what I know now. I always considered my self pretty healthy.

I used to work out at least five days a week, but usually six or seven. My diet was mostly chicken breast, brown rice, and vegetables. As far as nutrient density goes, based on what I know now, it was pretty bad. I ate low fat everything and relied mostly on hot sauce and spray butter to make my food palatable. Artificial sweeteners, energy drinks, seed oils, you name it: I was eating truckloads of that stuff. I even drank straight safflower oil. Oh and the supplements: anything that came in a powder and you could buy at GNC, you can bet I was on it.

Despite all that, I managed to stay pretty lean and pack on a great deal of muscle. When I finally got serious about working out, right after my senior year of high school, I was about 180 pounds and not very strong. Right before I started Paleo, I was around 245 pounds, 6'3", about 8% body fat, and could move some serious weight in the gym. So as you can see, the bodybuilding lifestyle had its rewards.

About two years ago, my roommates (Navy SEALs) started talking to me about diet. It was slow at first, just throwing stuff out at me and seeing what I had to say. Then one of my roommates presented me with *Good Calories, Bad Calories*, by Gary Taubes. It was a tough read and I got burned out on it pretty quickly, but it sparked my interest. Then I read *Primal Body, Primal Mind* by Nora Gegaudas. That's when everything changed. I really couldn't believe the things she asserted in that book. It went against everything I knew. So I started doing more research and reading more books and I haven't looked back since. Sure, I'm still set in my "bodybuilding" ways - and my performance in the gym will always come before anything else, - but I was 31 years old and I needed to start thinking about my long term health.

My girlfriend had done a few figure competitions and was a dedicated gym rat as well. However she had some health issues that just wouldn't go away. She always had trouble leaning out, was usually bloated, had frequent acne breakouts, and her menstrual cycle wreaked havoc on her body and on my sanity. I started to tell her about what I was reading, and we slowly started to figure that she has a gluten intolerance. Dairy seemed to be a problem for her as well.

The two of us made the choice to go "paleo" together. Let me tell you, if you're going to go Paleo, it's a hell of a lot easier if your spouse/significant other is willing to do it with you. At first we were pretty strict, following a strict program called Whole 30. We were very low carbohydrate – as was the bulk of the paleo community at the time. The switch was pretty easy for me, because I had been following some form of diet over the prior 15 years. I had a lot of cravings at first but, coming from the bodybuilding background, I was no stranger to cravings or hunger, so it didn't bother me. I felt great. I had tons of energy, I stopped taking naps, I quit most of the supplements I was on, and I even quit drinking coffee because I just didn't need it. I started to lean out even and I dropped to around 230 pounds. The only problem I had was that some of this weight loss was muscle. I also noticed it starting to affect my performance in the gym. I was losing muscle and getting weaker. I just couldn't keep working out like I used to as the low carb had me seriously burnt out, and I knew something had to change. I tried to get into ketosis a few times thinking that might help, not touching carbs for weeks at a time, but I don't think it ever really happened due to my high protein intake. So there I was again, self-experimentation and trial and error.

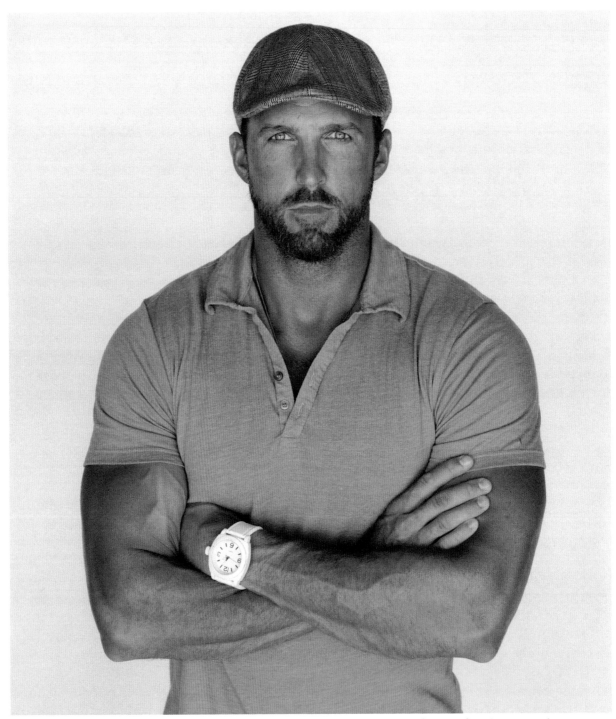

I came to a realization that my battle was no longer the choice of what foods to eat, but whether those foods (paleo foods) would support my bodybuilding lifestyle - if not, could I deal with that because the benefits were too great. The conclusion I came to was: Yes and No.

I was going to have to make some sacrifices to my bodybuilding progress if I was going to be paleo. I would probably not be as big and lean as I was pre-paleo but, in exchange, I would feel better and overall be healthier. Although I knew I would choose to be paleo, it was still a tough choice to make.

Sometimes I wished I would have just taken the blue pill.

Luckily the paleo community started to turn around on the subject of whether carbohydrates were good. When you haven't had them for a significant period of time, carbohydrates taste like heaven. Suddenly my workouts were back on track. I modified my workouts and went down the road of Powerlifting. This decreased my workload quite a bit, while allowing my strength levels to go through the roof.

Now I'm back up to about 235-240 pounds and stronger than I've ever been. I carry a little more body fat than I used to, but I've realized that comes with the increased performance. I'm now steadily rebuilding and although I've modified the Paleo template to meet my goals, I know that I've made the right decision.

My personal fitness has always been a two steps forward, one step back process. I definitely needed to take a step back and figure out what was really important and why I was even doing all this. I love working out and it is a huge part of my life, and I still want to be working out when I'm 50, 60, or even 70 years old. So I needed to make some changes. No more "dieting" in the common sense of the word: With paleo, I now have an eating plan for the rest of my life.

CHRISTINA LIANOS

NEW YORK CITY, NEW YORK

I truly don't recall a time in my life where I could tell you "I FEEL GREAT!" There was always a lingering cold, irritating and constant throat clearing, dull body aches, joint pain, muscle stiffness, daily headaches, debilitating migraines, uterine cramps, achy arches, joints, neck, back, gastric distress, abdominal bloating, severe PMS, a weakened immune system, thinning hair, brittle nails, dry skin, cold hands and feet, plantar fasciitis, insomnia or restless sleep, overall fatigue, keratosis pilaris, brain fog and a slew of other ailments - none of which seemed to be of any critical concern to the many medical professionals treating me over the years.

And then there was a long history of medical procedures and surgeries: a long battle with recurring pneumonia and upper respiratory issues at age 7 that resulted in routine radiology and numerous procedures that culminated in a lung removal at age 9; mysterious oral, nasal, and ocular ulcerations that plagued me through my teens into early adulthood before I was diagnosed with Behçet's Syndrome; I had multiple cysts drained and fibro adenoma tumors removed from both my breasts in my early 20s; all out breast surgery at 27; diagnosed with clinical "depression" in my early 30s followed by a Hashimoto Thyroiditis diagnosis for my 40th birthday. Lucky me!

I am fortunate to be alive, of that I am sure. And the realization that mid-life was not going to bring any improvements to my health and physical appearance shook me out of my complacency. As an obstinate force of nature, I became resolutely determined NOT to let what everyone had told me about the downward rickety spiraling of turning 40. I am a modern woman, a she-warrior, with a load of life left. That, coupled with a bit of internal vanity, a whole lot of anger, and an intense drive to prove people wrong, I decided to get smart and eventually found my way to paleo. This survivor was NOT going to let the next phase of my life roll downhill without a fierce fight.

Growing up in a Greek family, we naturally ate fresh fruits and vegetables, olive oil, meats, and fish. Very minimal processed foods were allowed into the house. Eating out was rare and I don't ever recall an overabundance of pasta or wheat in the house – other than bread. Moving out gave me freedom to rebel and eat things we weren't exposed to as kids. My pre-paleo diet was for the most part a SAD diet and my plate adhered to the USDA recommendations of fruits, vegetables, "heart healthy whole grains", lean proteins, and super low fats. Little did I realize I was starving myself, destroying my metabolism, and creating the perfect breeding ground for a host of health problems. Why would I ever question anything or anyone? "They" knew what they were talking about. Right?

So gravely and abysmally wrong.

October 2009, I was turning 40 and I was a literal medical and mental mess. I blamed my newly diagnosed hypothyroid condition as the cause of my weight gain and my weight gain for the cause of my deeper depression. I had always questioned my doctors about how my two pregnancies could both result in improved overall health and weight loss. I never gained more than 5-10 pounds, and my post-birth weight was both times less than pre-pregnancy. But they had no meaningful answers. I am not sure why I figured "they" had to know more than me. It never occurred to me that "they" could have had it all wrong.

So, armed with my Synthroid and Wellbutrin, I ventured into the abyss, believing that the weight would come off, I would be happier, that my body would positively respond and my energy would increase. What followed was almost 2 years of massive mood swings, weight fluctuations, deeper pain and an irrational anger that ushered in what were quite possibly the darkest days of my life.

In 2010, at 5', 7", and now a mortifying 190 pounds, I stopped stepping on the scale and stopped looking in the mirror. I truly did not know how to deal with my situation any longer. The weight may have gone up and down but I didn't want to know anymore. It was a losing battle that consumed my every thought and emotion.

It wasn't until the fall of 2010 that I started researching Hashimoto's and read about the link between it and gluten. I immediately gave up wheat and started feeling energy improvements within a month. But as with typical Hashi's, the symptoms starting returning among other new symptoms. The typical medical response? Increase dosage and take additional prescription drugs...the medical industry and pharmaceutical companies had created a lifetime client in me.

But I refused to be a sucker this time. I started to delve into all the available information about thyroid disorders. The more questions I asked, the more questions were raised. I started to have serious doubts about the course of treatment I was prescribed as well as the validity of everything any medical professional was telling me. My medical anomalies were never considered in their totality, and I was brushed off with a "you just have to eat less and exercise more." WTF?!? I was barely allowing myself to consume more than 1,200 calories a day and there was never a significant change in my weight with or without a fitness routine.

By the spring of 2011, a new doctor was diligent enough to dig deeper and test all of my vitamin and mineral levels. He found my vitamin D levels almost non-existent, and my B-12 and DHEA grossly deficient. Not surprisingly, cortisol was elevated too. A few months into supplementation I started to feel better. I stopped taking antidepressants and fairly quickly noticed some of the dark clouds lift.

Already gluten free, I had heard about the paleo lifestyle through my friend Laurie. I was inspired by her leap of faith and the amazing results I witnessed her achieve. I jumped on board and quickly committed to eliminating all grains.

The problem was, the concept never fully clicked. I was allowing myself offending foods here and there, constantly rationalizing "How can one slice of pizza hurt me if I only indulge once every so often?" I had yet to understand the power of food – that I was feeding the disease – and it had to stop.

In mid-October 2011, a year before the writing of this, I lost complete control of my anger. I was raging frequently over the smallest things. I was experiencing stroke-like episodes after massive fits of rage, and even became profoundly worried that I would need to be committed. My kids were in constant fear of something happening to me. My husband was at his wits end and trying to determine how he was going to minimize the damage should something unthinkable happen. Hundreds of miles away from any family, I was alone, afraid and severely unable to cope. While I managed to keep it together in public, home became hell.

On my 42nd birthday, broken, middle aged, fat, aging and tired of it all, I finally connected the dots. It occurred to me that the raging started 2 months into taking Armour and while it has worked so well for so many, it was clearly the wrong medication for me. I stopped taking it immediately and put all my efforts into healing my body naturally from the inside out. I had amassed hundreds of hours of research and concluded that I had no other alternative. It was either this, or sentencing myself to a miserable quality of life.

Enter paleo. Again. The idea of "diet" and the consuming thoughts of weight loss were banished from my mind and I ushered in a new era of self-awareness. I listened to my body for the first time. I started to eat full breakfasts, with lots of protein cooked in butter or coconut oil, served with a side of bacon. I thought I had died and gone to heaven those first few weeks of glorious indulgence.

I started to eat full lunches with clean vegetables, good quality protein, and MORE fat. No more rationing, no measuring, no concern over portion control, just eating clean. Dinner was the same. My body responded positively and I never overate, nor did I ever feel hungry. I never felt deprived nor did I crave junk. And I didn't gain an ounce. In fact, I lost a few pounds and proceeded to lose more weight every week.

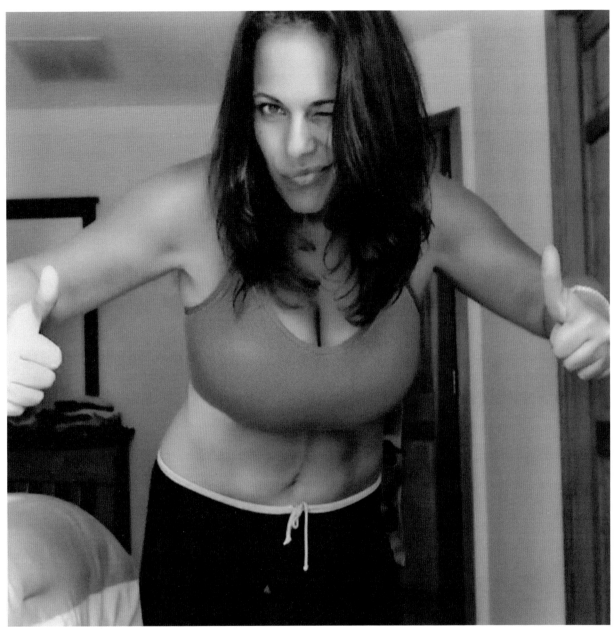

Within two months, all the pains, aches, headaches, backaches … everything I outlined previously … WERE GONE. I was in utter disbelief. Two decades had elapsed, and there was not one day without a headache. By contrast I was now pain free for weeks.

Sometimes we slip up, because we are human. And I slipped up hard during the holidays where a few indulgences here and there led to more indulgences and eventually a massive weight jump. The floodgate of symptoms opened and crashed upon me fiercely. I turned my feeling of defeat, self-loathing and guilt into motivation to commit 100% to the paleo lifestyle.

January 1st, 2012 was the first day of my rebirth. No grains, no sugar, and minimal dairy. As of today, I am virtually symptom-free. I feel better and stronger in my 40s than I ever did in my 20s. I am holding steady at 155 pounds and though I want to see the scale decrease a bit more, I am no longer a slave to those numbers. I fit into clothing I wore 15 years ago when I was 20 pounds lighter. I have lost more than 4 inches from my waist, 2 band sizes, 2 inches from my hips, and a whopping 3 inches off my thighs.

My skin has aged well and I have managed to keep those first wrinkles I noticed on my 40th birthday at bay. My thinning hair is thickening and I cannot keep up with nail growth.

My favorite improvement has been the new relationship I have formed with my body. It talks to me. I listen. I nourish it. It performs for me. My body is now stronger, more resilient and far more capable of doing more physical exercise.

Miraculously, I no longer crave junk. I can pass by a bakery or a pizzeria and not be besieged by the desire to dive face first into a pie or devour an entire loaf of bread. I feel no need to eat unacceptable food when there are no alternatives. My body is well adapted and can fast for long periods of time if needed, without any insulin spikes.

My nuggets of wisdom? Love yourself first. Accept your body and embrace what it can and cannot do for you. It's the only one you have and it's up to you to worship it. Nourish it properly and it will talk to you, reward you with better physical and mental health. That bread you gave up to get fit and healthy? Leave it in the past. Don't try to fake it with paleo ingredients. Shift your focus and your thinking to the many wonderful things you can eat and the rest will follow.

Paleo is a way of life. We are all very much works in progress, recovering from years of doing it wrong. I have learned to look beyond the result and appreciate my paleo journey to optimal health as the ultimate goal. And I can now happily report that ... I FEEL GREAT!

MICHELLE ALEXANDRA STUPAY

AUBURN, ALABAMA

mas0046@auburn.edu

There is a lot to be said about paleo and it's effects on your body. It's definitely interesting to look at my body now and compare it to my body six months ago, and even a year ago. One year ago I weighed approximately 150 pounds, maybe 148, on a good day, whereas today I weigh 155 pounds...but I look completely different. The shape of my face is completely different, clothes fit differently, and my mind has made a total 180 degree turn. Here's the irony: These days I might work out 3 days a week, I eat more than most people should, and can even enjoy a college weekend without guilt. So it is very interesting to me, indeed, that changing my diet has actually completely changed my life. I don't mean change my life in the "I lost 100+ pounds," or "my diabetes is gone," which are both great accomplishments, but it changed my way of thinking. Paleo has allowed me to learn to enjoy life, instead of worrying about calories, feeling guilty over what I ate, avoiding social situations that provided temptation that could "throw me off," and driving myself absolutely insane over everything (which drove me to the verge of depression, caused me to form a little Body Dysmorphic Disorder and, at my lowest point, slight purging tendencies). I am now able to go to dinner with friends, have drinks, and enjoy everything I do. Paleo truly saved me from myself.

I was 138 pounds in September of 2010, the beginning of freshman year. I was healthy, with no chronic diseases or issues, and was highly active. I ate the typical high-carb, low-fat American diet and allowed myself to enjoy weekends with a less optimal diet. I went on birth control that September when I started college (one can never be too cautious) and despite my relatively "healthy" eating habits and 6 days a week of workouts, I steadily gained 12 pounds. So there I was, 150 pounds of miserable freshman on the floor of the dorm, crying to my sister on the phone, who suggested this paleo way of eating which her boyfriend advocated. A week later, I moved out of the dorms into my own place and began my journey.

If there is one thing I love, it's bacon. I could eat it all day, every day. So when someone suggested that I can eat as much of it as I wanted….well, you get the picture. Shortly after starting paleo, I began crossfitting. I fell in love with the combination. I was able to workout, which I absolutely love to do, and eat more food...what else could I ask for? As I began becoming more and more accustomed to this new lifestyle, I realized I had not lost weight and I slowly became obsessed with my caloric intake. I felt great, but wasn't happy with what I saw. After my freshman year, I had low self-esteem and low self-confidence, which was very unlike me. The mental aspect of paleo was the hardest part of the switch for me, not the dietary changes. I cut the grains, most sugar, most dairy, and as much processed food I could. So there I was making this huge change that was supposed to make me lose weight - and I was failing at it. As a result, I began messing with macro ratios, fasting, working out two and three times a day, five days a week, super calorie restriction, and anything else. I was on an out of control "paleo" Yo-Yo diet. Some weeks I would be super strict, others I would be more slack with what I ate but restrict myself calorie-wise, and, eventually, I would break and binge on things like cake and ice cream. I slowly began to spiral out of control.

By January of 2012 I was avoiding going out with my friends because I would end up staring at myself in the mirror, poking at fat, grabbing parts of my body I hated, and crying. Although I may have been following paleo eating guidelines, I wasn't living the paleo lifestyle. If you talk to anyone about paleo, they will say you should not let what you eat control you, and that you should be able to enjoy your life, be stress free, and enjoy all the benefits that go with that.

In February, I hurt my back. Overtraining became impossible as I began to back off from my workouts due to excruciating pain. I am a super-competitive person, and removing myself from the crossfit gym was the first step on my road to "recovery." I began lifting three days a week, fasting, while tracking my food and calories. Although I was not rid of my neuroticism, this was the first time I felt like I had some control over what I was doing. I began feeling happier and looking better. Although I was a strong 155 pounds when I first hurt myself, I didn't look like the athlete that I was. Training two and three times a day put me in great shape, but my body couldn't handle the stress. I developed that "spare tire" we all know and love. The goal was to get rid of it, but no matter what I did it would not go away. Then I realized that less is more.

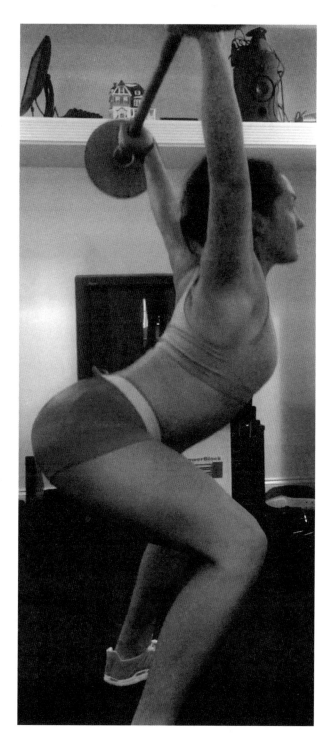

Since my first back injury in February I have been sick multiple times and re-injured my back. I eventually took off 8 weeks between mid-June and mid-August; focusing on eating well, lots of low intensity exercise (walking, swimming, yoga, etc.), getting enough rest, enjoying friends and family, and just being happy. These are the staples of the paleo lifestyle. And although my weight has yet to decline from 155, I have been able to start working out again (only 3 days a week now), and have returned to school a completely different person. After I adapted all aspects of the paleo lifestyle, eating and otherwise, and applied them to everyday life, I have seen a complete shift in both my mindset and my body. The person I am now and the person I was before are two completely different people. My mood has improved, and self-confidence and self-esteem have increased. My body is beginning to change for the better, and my quality of life has improved so much I can't help but to smile every day. This is not something I would have been able to do alone. I had the support of quite a few people from the *International Paleo Movement Group*, a group on Facebook (http://is.gd/ paleogroup), who helped me solve my problems through their constant questioning, sharing, research, tomfoolery, and "food porn" pictures. I learned a lot and made many great connections, and continue to do so on a daily basis.

While I do occasionally cheat on my diet, the mental ability to not feel guilt and enjoy these special occasions is an amazing breakthrough for me. It was not until I fully grasped paleo, in all aspects of the lifestyle, that I was able to save myself from my self-destructive tendencies. I am finally able to enjoy my time in college to the fullest, and plan to enjoy the rest of my life paleo as fu#k.

EVE HAAPALA

TALLINN, ESTONIA

theprimalwoman.blogspot.com

My childhood was an extremely happy one – I grew up enjoying the freedom of true country living – spending my days with my two best friends roaming the nearby woods, fishing, running, playing barefoot in the open air. Even the cold and snowy northern winter days were spent outside from dawn till dusk or later, after school hours.

In my early teens things started changing. I started to experience allergies and sensitivities, and I started to put on weight. Nothing that concerned me – maybe 6-9 pounds extra. I decided to lose weight for my high school graduation. At that age we all deal with peer pressure, and so did I. Therefore I decided to go vegan as all of my closest friends were doing it, and they all were skinny and gorgeous. After about 6 months so was I – I weighed at my lowest around 106 pounds at 5', 6" tall. But my health was getting worse and worse. I was suffering from continuous colds. In the spring of 1998, just before graduation, I had a series of angina and laryngitis that killed my voice – I was a promising singer (classical) before that – and this loss still hurts deeply. After graduation, I luckily came to my senses. I was simply too physically and mentally fatigued to continue with veganism and with the disbanding of my vegan friends, each going a separate way with their lives, I went back to eating "normally" again. I was also (mis)diagnosed as being "allergic" to gluten at the age of 13, and I had been following the doctor's orders to ingest small amount of gluten continuously in order to desensitize myself to it. I later learned I had celiac disease.

I got a little better before getting a lot worse.

It was a gorgeous day in early May 2001. My 21st birthday was nearing and I was on the top of the world – studying what I was passionate about in the best university in the country. I had found the most wonderful friends and I had just bought my own flat in a beautiful neighborhood. In addition to all that, I also happened to be in love. That day I went to see my doctor about a curious numbness in my right quad. I thought it was a case of DOMS (delayed onset muscle soreness) gone wrong. I got the shock of my life finding out that it wasn´t. Instead of going home with a prescription for the usual 800mg ibuprofen, I was promptly sent to ENMG (electroneuromyography), and given an MRI and lumbar puncture. The diagnosis didn't take too long, but the wait, I admit, was unnerving. When the results came, I was called in for a private meeting with my doctor, who explained, holding my hand, that I had MS. Multiple Sclerosis. I left that office with a pile of papers with prescriptions for several different drugs and a cocktail of 6 antidepressants and a prognosis of maximum 10 years until a lifetime spent in a wheelchair.

I never took the drugs. Not one of them.

My life changed completely that day. I changed the course of my studies to better understand my prognosis, and minored in molecular biology and biochemistry with an emphasis in evolution because it became more and more evident that I wouldn't get anything useful out of my doctors - besides writing a prescription – or ten. I spent all my free time studying this disease and alienated my friends, family, and finally also my boyfriend, who probably was more scared of the possible outcome of this condition than I was. But I was certain of one thing – there had to be a reason out there, and an explanation – my faith in science was formidable indeed. And I decided that I was going to dig the answer up.

In 2001, in an ex-soviet country, internet access to peer-reviewed (or otherwise) international studies was not as excellent as it is now. It was a whole different world 10 years ago. But there were some sparks in the darkness – a few blogs here and there. So, quite soon after embarking on my quest of knowledge that year, I came across Arthur DeVany's Evolutionary Fitness blog. I'm not certain it was even called that back then. At that point all I had studied, and feared, suddenly made sense. The connection between my celiac disease and MS made sense. The evolutionary background behind autoimmune responses, the whole mechanism of protection gone wrong and why it happens, became clear to me. At that point the term "paleo" wasn't coined yet. Lauren Cordain's *The Paleo Diet* had yet to be published.

Now I understood that I had been killing myself slowly, and I decided to experiment with going mostly gluten free. Reading Weston A. Price's *Nutrition and Physical Degeneration* was probably the biggest motivating factor for me to make that change. In the spirit of Weston Price, I tried everything to simulate my "traditional diet" – sprouting my grains and baking sourdough bread. The problem was that even though my symptoms became much less dominant, they were still there. Regressions still happened. It took me almost a year of self experimentation to finally fully give up gluten bearing grains – but even that didn't "cure" me.

Year 2003 brought a new blog into existence – Mark Sisson's Mark's Daily Apple. From there on my eyes finally really opened and the evolutionary biology + biochemistry + epigenetics clicked in my head and I understood that the name of the cereal protein doesn't matter – its action does –and their actions are all the same. So I ditched all grains in 2003 – and everything else that might promote inflammation: processed foods, low-fat processed dairy,

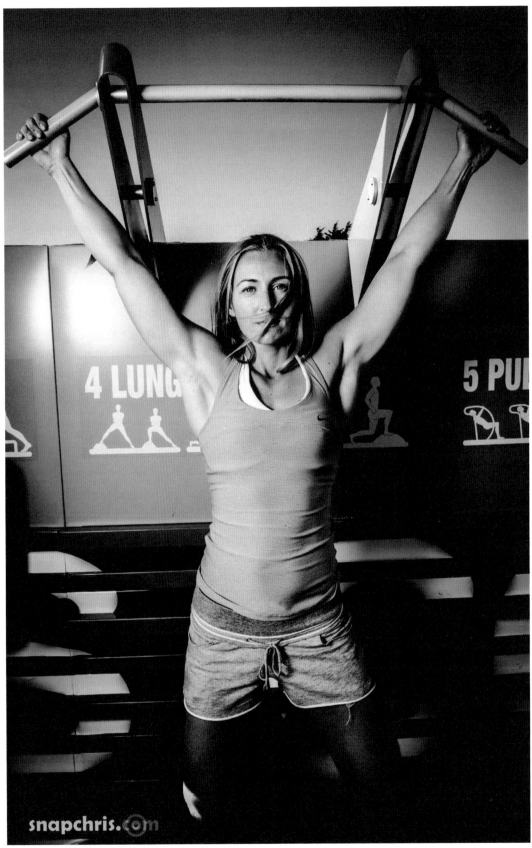

(photo by Chris Willis, www.snapchris.com)

nuts, seeds, seed oils, fructose, and nightshades.

Hey, I just realized, my paleo 10-year anniversary is coming up! I feel like I owe my life to Devany's Evolutionary Fitness, and he is a man I will always have infinite respect for. But it is the paleo lifestyle in its totality that got me where I am now. I am completely healthy and very fit. I began to lift weights and became a competitive power lifter and long-distance cyclist. Although I'm not competing any longer, I still work out and enjoy doing it. When I say "the Paleo lifestyle" I mean that for me it is so much more than just a diet or a way of eating. For me it means living a simpler life overall – avoiding stress, taking things slowly, enjoying the moment and taking time to take care of myself. Living a more "physical" life – using your body in the way it was meant to be used – to haul heavy things, sprint fast once in a while, and walk as much as possible. In addition to that, living a more "pure" life - avoiding chemicals wherever possible and preferring natural skin/hair care, personal hygiene, and home cleaning products. As a combined result of all that – a complete paleo lifestyle – I have been lesion-free for the last seven years. And I can safely say that my future will not be spent in a wheelchair.

TONY KASANDRINOS

FORTH WORTH, TEXAS

www.kasandrinos.com

I first learned about paleo when I was training at Crossfit Center City (CFCC) in Philadelphia, Pennsylvania, back in 2010. I had been training for about 6 months and felt great, but still had about 5-10 pounds of body fat I wanted to lose. I have never been overweight and never really felt too bad after I ate. I have been in the military for 15 years and prior to that was very involved in football, boxing, and track. I was eating ok (a lot of meat and vegetables, but would still have the occasional pizza, Philly Cheese steak, and lots of bread on the side).

Then Greg Privitera and Erin Davidson decided to do a body composition challenge for all the CFCC members. That's when I really learned about what paleo was. So I started doing a little research. We did track our macronutrients (fat, protein, carbs), but really focused on eating paleo foods. For the first time in my life I was eating A LOT of vegetables. I always loved eating animal meat, so that was not an issue. I soon discovered some amazing websites that I still follow today (like Balancedbites.com and Marksdailyapple.com). Over the course of that 30-day challenge, I lost about 2 inches off my waist, about 8 pounds, and felt much better all around. The changes I saw in myself and the people around me made me really get interested in what food does to the body and how important it really is. I always thought you could out train a bad diet - but then again I always thought pasta and bread were healthy for you.

Fast forward a year: I was training pretty hard at crossfit, eating about 80-90% paleo, cheating here and there with a beer or dessert. I was feeling pretty good and hovered around 12-14% body fat. Now it was time for my one week seminar with MOVNAT in West Virginia. During that week we moved most of the day and got a large amount of rest. We also ate 100% paleo. Not a single cheat. I can honestly say, when I ate 100% with not a single cheat, I have never felt better. It is not always easy in everyday life to eat totally clean (100% paleo), especially if you are not cooking all your food. Even if you think you are eating right when eating out, there is often cross contamination with gluten. A few weeks after getting back from MOVNAT I went to Greece for an entire month. I spent that entire month eating fresh animals, fish, and vegetables (and an inordinate amount of figs, lol). Being away from America and focusing on QUALITY paleo food changed everything for me. I actually paid attention to the fact that the fish I ate was not farm raised. The lamb I ate for dinner was raised on the food the mountains provided it - not an artificial diet full of grains or corn designed to fatten it up. The chicken we ate was in the backyard eating bugs, fruit, and snakes (YES THEY EAT SNAKES) - it's natural, species-appropriate food - as opposed to the soy and vegetarian diets that the chickens you buy in the store are fed. This was the first time I really thought about what the animals eat. It makes so much sense when you think about it - but unfortunately it is something most people do not think about.

After that summer I became much more concerned with where our food comes from. I am to the point now where I don't want to eat any animals that are not being raised properly. I try to always use local farmers. My paleo journey began with cutting out pasta and gluten and eating meat and vegetables. Now I am focusing on not only eating "paleo foods" but also focusing on where that food comes from and what my food ate while it was alive.

Likewise, I have also become more concerned with finding quality fats to cook with. For example, there are few standards on regulating olive oil and 69% of imported olive oils failed to meet even those standards - because they are mixed with low quality seed and other oils. People should know that the olive oil they are buying is really 100% olive oil - despite the deceptive labeling that pervades the industry. As a result, since becoming paleo, I have gotten much more involved with my family's olive oil importing business. Check out myfamily's website if you want to know more: www.kasandrinos.com .

I conclude with this: Is it easier to just eat a SAD diet? Yes it is. Is it worth the time, money, and effort in eating a true paleo diet? HELL YES!!!!

DAVID

GAINESVILLE, FLORIDA

On November 17, 1999 I was diagnosed with Embryonal Carcinoma Stage 2. I underwent two surgeries. Initially, I went in for a biopsy of the tumor, and once the doctor determined that it was malignant, they amputated the right testicle and vas deferens. The next surgery came when I had an intravenous port placed under my skin just below the left clavicle bone. The line was inserted into my clavicle vein, allowing the chemo drugs to be pumped directly into my heart, allowing the heart to evenly distribute them to my body. The best way I can describe how that felt was the feeling of a constant bee stinging that area of my chest. I went through 4 chemo sessions over a three month period. I would check into the hospital on Sunday evening, get hooked up to the IV and then they would begin my 9 hour a day drip on Monday morning. I would be up again by 8am first for anti-nausea meds. Then I would get a 5 hour drip of Cisplatin, followed by a saline flush of my chest, then a 3 hour drip of Etoposide, followed by another saline flush. I would do this for five consecutive days, once every three weeks. I lost all of my hair from head to toe. I had to walk around in public with a sanitary mask on to avoid contact with germs because of my weakened immune system.

There were some side effects that lingered for years following the chemo. Most notably, often times after eating, I would get shooting pains in the upper left of my chest. Sometimes, they came on so swift and hard that I would get dizzy and think I was having a heart attack (in my 20s…yeah). I went to my doctor and she could not figure it out. I went to a neurologist because I thought maybe it was nerve damage from the port. Nope. I went to a cardiologist to see if I really had a heart complication. Nothing there either. It had been written off as something I would just have to deal with. I never was given any meds because nothing was determined as a cause or symptom to treat.

I tried several different diets over the course of a few years. I'd lose a little weight, get bored with it and gain it back. Nothing ever seemed to work for any length of time. I even tried going vegetarian for a couple of weeks.

Typically, I ate a bowl of cereal or bagels or some other similar breakfast food. Lunch was either leftovers or take out, usually with a big helping of pasta, rice or bread. Dinner was more of the same, a meat, a cooked, previously frozen veggie and loads of rice, pasta or other breads with sauces or toppings galore. All followed by some ice cream typically. Mostly, I tried to maintain low-fat and high carb.

My overall health pre-paleo was bad, but it would have definitely become a lot worse had I not discovered paleo. I used to smoke about 1.5 packs of Winston 100's every day. I didn't do any activities outside of working - except maybe some yard work for a couple of hours a week.

Leading up to my paleo switch in February of 2011, I was 29 years old and 270 pounds. I had become frustrated with the fact that I could not keep up with my two young boys, my relationship with my wife was losing steam, and I was constantly overstressed over anything and everything.

One day, my oldest son came up to me while I was eating dinner and said "Daddy, you must be able to eat a lot of food." I asked him what made him want to say that. He says to me, "Because you have such a big belly, you must be able to eat more than anyone else ever!" Kids certainly have a way with words…suffice to say, it was time for a change.

Vegetarianism is what led me to the Paleo Lifestyle. I picked up and read a book called "The China Study," also known as The Vegetarian's Bible. Then I discovered countless articles debunking the book online, like Denise Minger's at http://rawfoodsos.com/the-china-study . I eventually stumbled upon an author named Robb Wolf and his book "The Paleo Solution." I read about his journey through vegetarianism and how his path brought him to the paleo lifestyle. Then I decided to try it. What could it hurt? I had tried the Weight Watchers thing, vegetarian thing, tried eating smaller portions of the same SAD foods, and even eliminated fast foods and sodas with little success. I was tracking and obsessing over every detail in a website called myfitnesspal.com, measuring every calorie I was consuming.

On February 6th, 2011 I quit smoking cold turkey for about the 14th time. I was determined to quit and improve because of what my son had said. With the help of my family and friends holding me accountable all day long via Facebook, it stuck this time. And In May of 2011, I made the switch to paleo. And I have never looked back.

The switch was relatively easy for me. I gave up dairy first because I didn't care for it either way. Then I gave up the grains and pastas. This was a problem for me because I come from a large Italian family and pasta is about as vital to life as breathing. It stayed a problem for several weeks until I realized that my chest pains were gone! So I experimented - after 8 weeks of no breads, I made a nice Italian style meal for my family. Before I got to the cannoli, the stabbing feeling in my chest returned. For two weeks after that I stayed away again. And there was no pain. I tried to eat a little pasta at my grandmother's house. Result: pain. I thought back to everything I had read, and words like Gluten Intolerance, Inflammation, and Anti-Nutrients kept coming through loud and clear. Although I have never been to a doctor to determine if I do have gluten intolerance, by my own process of elimination, I decided that I should avoid wheat, breads, rice, pasta and other gluten sources permanently.

I am now an avid bicyclist, commuting to work 12 miles each way, 2-3 times per week, often joining many other cyclists for fun and challenging group rides around the county roads. I also lift weights and I train for multiple sports. One of my goals now is to complete an Ironman before I turn 40, on a 100% paleo diet. My weight went from 270 pounds with a 44" waist to 182 pounds with a 32" waist. I was uncomfortable at the lower weight, and have since found balance with my body at about 195 pounds. I am 5',11" tall and still have a 32" waist. I no longer have pain in my chest after a meal, no matter how big it is. I have also cleared my seasonal allergies. I maintain a level of energy I don't think I have ever known – and it lasts all day long. I no longer have energy spikes and crashes throughout the day.

I recently had a physical exam with my doctor. When I described how the changes had helped me with all of these past issues, I was floored by what she told me. No congratulations, you look great, keep up the good work, your blood panels look fantastic, nothing. Instead, at 30 years old, she told me that if I kept eating this way, I would have to consider the fact that I will be on statins to avoid a heart attack within a couple of years. Unfortunately her opinion was not supported by the facts: my blood panels and CT screenings had never looked better in my life. I asked her why she thought that. She told me that the high levels of fat and protein in my diet were going to clog my arteries and put me at risk for attack or stroke. I asked her to elaborate how that works. She said that all the fat and grease goes straight into the blood stream and grabs onto the arterial walls. That's what fats do. I asked her why our cell structure and brain function require healthy doses of fat to function properly every day. She told me they don't and that they function perfectly fine on carbs and sugars. I asked her then about why, with the steady increase of sugars and carbohydrates in the SAD over the last few decades, the rate of heart disease and other "diseases of civilization" continue to grow rapidly and have begun to show up in children. She said that she didn't have an answer for that because she was not a nutritionist.

I left her office and vowed to never use her services again. I am currently looking for a new doctor in my town. I want a doctor that is interested in working with me in preventive

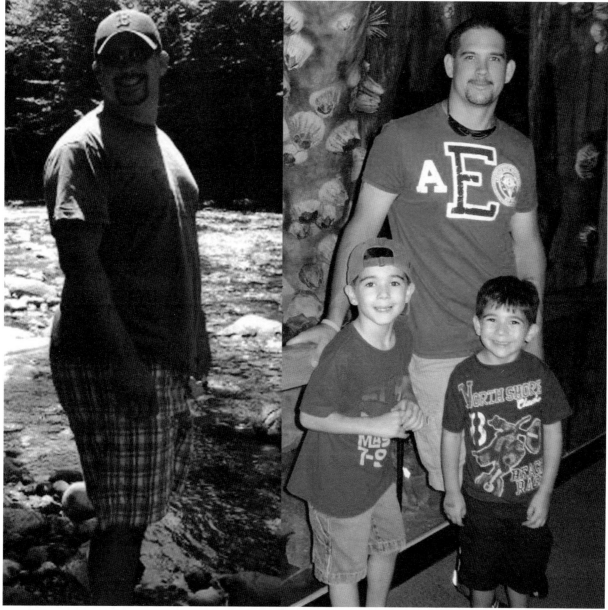

medicine via nutrition, exercise and a healthy lifestyle, not one who would just assume I am going to need statins soon based on what she was taught – and is unwilling to even consider that there is a problem with the dominant paradigm.

MONIQUE ALLEN

VACAVILLE, CALIFORNIA

moallen01@gmail.com

As someone who loves to eat and never tends to miss a meal, I have always struggled with my over indulgent personality when it comes to food. Add in the issue of having a kidney disease which required me to take steroids (like prednisone) and it makes for an explosive combination – and makes it exceptionally hard to remain healthy and fit. I am a 41 year old female, 5', 1", and I was weighing in at 183 pounds! Yikes! Something had to give. Even though I was exercising it still wasn't helping me lose weight because of foods that I was consuming.

Then a friend by the name of Joe Salama began touting the benefits of paleo on his Facebook page. Joe started posting all these delicious looking meals he was creating while discussing his life-changing benefits. Of course anything involving food automatically captures my interest. I was thinking the meals look so delish, it was tantamount to food porn at its finest… but it was HEALTHY!!!

I wanted to know more, so I emailed Joe about paleo and I started doing some research into the nutritional changes it would involve. I'll be honest, I had some doubts. I was worried that the consumption of all that protein would affect my kidneys. Doctors always steered me towards low-protein diets, and I even went so far as to become a vegan during my college years to manage my disease.

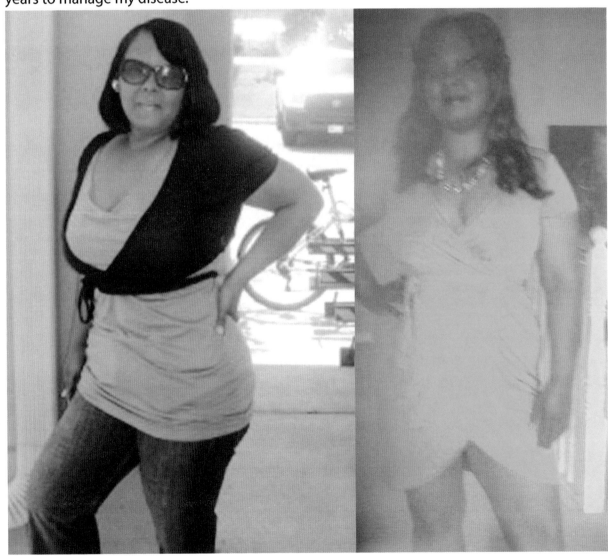

I decided to give paleo a try earlier this year. I told myself "OK let's try it for a couple of weeks, what's the harm?" I was shocked and amazed by how my body responded to the nutritional changes. I was more energetic. I actually stopped spilling protein (part of the kidney disease) and had some lab work done to assess the impact of the change. I still don't understand why paleo is reversing the protein spilling since doctors have always suggested I needed to *limit* my protein. But it works. And you can't argue with that.

Was it easy to become paleo? Absolutely NOT!!! You are talking about someone who loves to eat, cook, dine out, and review restaurants. I had to make the change in stages, and I am still working on eliminating some SAD habits but overall I am committed to seeing this through.

Since I have made some of the changes, I have lost a several inches around my belly and my fitness level has increased. I was discouraged initially because I was not seeing the pounds melt away despite that I FELT better. I stopped spilling protein in my urine and my energy level was great. Before making the switch, I would easily consume a significant amount of carbs from the bread I was eating. Desserts were a big issue for me, and I realized the sugar from the peach cobblers were literally toxic. Because of the health benefits that I have experienced, I know that paleo is not a fad, but it's a lifestyle where many rewards are reaped.

Although not everyone in my family is convinced that a high saturated fat diet is the best approach nutritionally, I have been able to get my mom to try paleo and she is now a believer! I remain committed to the lifestyle because it's the best health insurance plan I can vouch for at this time, and the results are simply incredible.

DANA MICHELLE NORRIS

AUSTIN, TEXAS

michelle@ancestralmomentum.com , www.instinctcatering.com

I've been paleo for about 7 years. I'm the Co-Owner & Executive Chef for Instinct Catering, Events & Supper Club in Austin, Texas as well as a Co-Founder and Partner of Paleo FX with my husband, Keith Norris.

Before I decided to change my lifestyle, I wasn't in poor health but I wasn't in optimum health, either. I did, however, suffer with being borderline celiac, and completely unaware of it. At 39 years of age, I weighed between 175 and 180 pounds. I worked out haphazardly. I would get a burst of inspiration and get on a workout kick and start "eating healthy" and lose 15 to 20 pounds, only to gain it back and yo-yo once more. Sound familiar? My specialty as a chef prior to going paleo was Italian, so we ate a lot of homemade pasta, bread, and pizza. I made fresh salads, vegetables and meats. I've not ever been one for processed foods, so there wasn't a big change for us there - but the bread, pasta, and sweets were toughest to give up. Imagine if you had a stomachache every time you ate; well, that was me. I suffered from IBS, Chronic Fatigue Syndrome, fibromyalgia, with severe migraines and daily throbbing dull headaches. The migraines and headaches were at times completely debilitating. I would be bedridden for days with a migraine and more often than not, it was accompanied by nausea and vomiting. At the time, I took three different preventive medications every day. I went in for cranial botox shots every two months. I took a medication for migraine onset to try to stave it off. Although it rarely worked, it was well worth those few times when it did. I also took one of two other medications for a full blown migraine, depending on whether it was accompanied by nausea or not. It seemed everything was a trigger for a migraine.

My husband Keith had been eating paleo for about a year, not eating any of my traditional Italian dishes when the family ate dinner. Before going paleo, he LOVED these dishes. When I questioned him and asked, "Are you really never going to have my pasta or pizza again?" He said, "No." Keith was not one to beat you over the head with anything, but every time my stomach hurt after eating, he would casually mention, "I really think you should get checked for celiac."

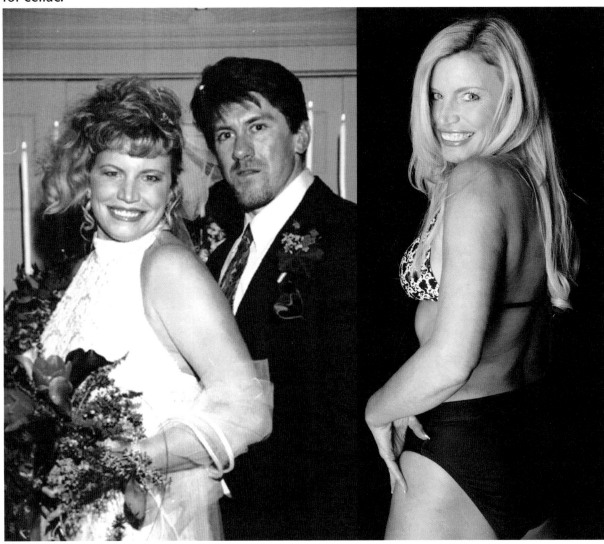

Well, one time he finally convinced me to look into it. I was tested for the anti-bodies and my test came back negative. I later learned that this was fairly typical. The doctor started discussing a biopsy of my colon and while he was explaining the procedure to me, he was literally falling asleep. I thought to myself: "There is no way I'm allowing him to cut into me!" I also was puzzled as to why this was the next step at all. Invasive surgery?!? Why wasn't that the last resort? It seemed far more intuitive to me to try eliminating the offensive foods from my diet and evaluating the effect of that before cutting someone up. So I opted to do that on my own.

Once I started eating paleo, my stomach aches, bloating (which I hadn't noticed until it was gone), IBS, chronic fatigue syndrome, and fibromyalgia all improved almost immediately. Also - something I wasn't even really aware of - my knees were swollen and ached a lot, and I had a dull ache in my lower back. I got used to the idea that I had some early form of arthritis in my joints – but once I went paleo, it was gone, completely gone. It's funny how things become "your normal" until you find out what "true normal" really is. I have since learned about the systemic inflammation that grains cause and in retrospect, the changes were a given. All these improvements were clearly noticeable at about the three weeks into eating paleo. The biggest and most amazing thing - something I never expected – was that my daily throbbing headaches disappeared. This has been the best improvement of all, a dramatic improvement to my quality of life. Imagine if you had a constant dull headache, all the time, and suddenly like that it was gone…Hallelujah!

It would take some time, but the migraines that had come at least once or twice a week are now under control and now I might get one once every six months if I am under a lot of stress. I do still take a preventative med, Flexeril, at the lowest dose possible, as a muscle relaxer. For full blown migraines I still take Imitrex, also the lowest dose. I anticipate being completely off of these meds within the next year.

I'm now 46, I eat a fairly strict paleo diet: I take heavy cream in my decaf coffee, I don't eat grains at all, and very little sugar. My sweets consist of fruits or small amounts of 85-90% dark chocolate, at most. I weigh between 130 and 135, and I exercise regularly training with my husband, Keith Norris of Efficient Exercise. We eat fresh meat or eggs and vegetables for almost every meal. We're very passionate about this lifestyle so we created our own website (www.ancestralmomentum.com). We feel so strongly about this lifestyle that we created the successful and popular Paleo FX Symposium (www.therealpaleofx.com). We hope to be able to bring this lifestyle to the masses - not only to bring about a healthier society, but to help combat our growing healthcare crisis. This is why we do what we do.

JAMIL MOLEDINA

SAN FRANCISCO, CALIFORNIA

twitter: @jmoledina

I usually roll my eyes at the mention of something that sounds like a fad diet. However, it seemed that I blindly stumbled into much of the paleo concept when implementing my own custom dietary plan. Sure, most health programs have obvious common factors, like eating less and exercising regularly, but the way to be successful seems to be what separates those that work from those that don't. By rolling my own, so to speak, I managed to lose 45 pounds in 4 months.

Two years ago, I decided to improve my health. I wanted to return to my law school dimensions for aesthetic reasons, but I also wanted to have the energy to chase down my increasingly boundary-pushing daughter. And of course, there was the connected interest in actually functioning effectively as a father long into the future. Once I set that specific metric

of law school measurements as a goal, I thought about how I got away from that condition. I had put on nearly fifty pounds over a decade and a bit, aided by cushy jobs, no exercise, and foodiness. I also thought about all the ways I had tried to lose weight in the past, which failed. At one point, I worked out hard for an hour at the gym every day for two weeks, saw no results, and then quit. I heard about Atkins, it sounded implausible, and never tried it. Another time, I tried to be a pesceterian, but that also had no effect. And so on and so forth. I had no real first hand proof that I could lose weight, but it had to happen. I had to find a way. I cleared my head, went back to fundamentals, and thought about what I remembered about human physiology, what should make sense. And I made a plan.

I live in the real world. I live my life, I enjoy life. Plus I'm not good with outright deprivation. The real magic was in translating my plan and my commitment to my goal into my life. As a first step, to prepare better food and add daily exercise, I needed to create more time in the day. So I canceled cable. Battlestar Galactica was over, so removing TV wasn't a big loss. In order to exercise the bare minimum to have a therapeutic effect, I decided to run 25-30 minutes every day. I had a treadmill, so that vastly cut the time wasted in getting to and from a gym near my home. I worked at Electronic Arts at the time, and the Club One gym at EA was right next to where I worked, so that was also an efficient option while at work. And the soccer field in one of the Mission neighborhood parks near my home was also a good option.

I picked running because it requires no other people or special equipment. You can do it anywhere, anytime, and even use it as a means of getting to places on time if you're running late. I didn't work out for a long time per session, or run particularly fast. I did run continuously. When at the gym, I would lift weights too. But really, it was never to the point where I became too exhausted to do it again the next day. But even so, those weren't a fun 30 minutes. To counteract the pain and boredom of exercise, I created classic sci-fi and fantasy movie soundtrack playlists. Basil Poledouris's iconic Conan the Barbarian score in particular has a great percussive hammer beat, that's ideal for a relaxed but continuous running pace. But my top recommendation is Don Davis's frantic score to The Matrix. You'll be reliving those scenes as if you had been sucked into the Matrix yourself, and before you know it, your 25,000 B.T.U.s of body heat will have been channeled productively.

I threw out all packaged and processed food from my home. I threw out all sweets and refined sugars. I only stocked natural foods, like nuts, fruits, and tuna steaks. Some grains remained, like pasta, but my consumption of them went down to 10% of my total meals. I could never cut it out entirely, it's my favorite food. Out in the commercial packaged food world, I bought things in the supermarket only if stocked around the perimeter – so that's dairy, meat, and produce. I ate raw fruits and vegetables for breakfast and dinner, and ate the normal entree portion of a lunch for lunch. EA's cafeteria was great for this normal lunch, since they served small portions of highly nutritious and tasty real food. Perfect for me. At conferences, my first stop would be a supermarket, and I'd fill my room with fruits and vegetables. I stopped drinking alcohol, and had water instead. I stopped drinking sugar-based beverages outright, they are just frivolous overhead calories. And because I'm not a monk, I had one splurge day every two weeks. On that day, I would eat a lot of good food all day, and allow myself one dessert and some drinks. For a man living a mostly austere food life, seeing me pig out at Stubbs BBQ was quite mind-blowing for some of my Austin friends.

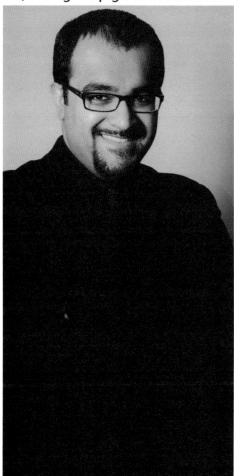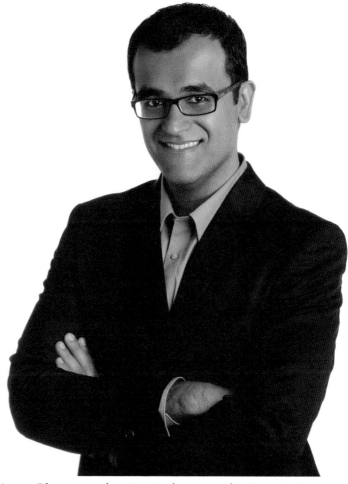

(2009 photo credit: Harry Lang, Harry Lang Photography; 2010 photo credit: Gene X Huang, Orange Photography)

Following this regimen, I lost 45 pounds over the course of a summer. I also happened to shave my goatee, and replace my entire wardrobe. At PAX, people didn't recognize me. It's not that I was particularly overweight to start with, but it was still startling to a lot of people. Internally, I felt like a new man. My little aches went away, and I felt much more alive. Only then did I read Michael Pollan's *The Omnivore's Dilemma*, Christopher MacDougall's *Born to Run*, and all the articles tying caloric restriction to rejuvenation. All of these sources validated my own regimen, all the way down to my running in those ugly but unpadded Vibram Five Fingers shoes. My friend Joe Salama discovered paleo after I got back in shape, and as we shared stories of our experiences, we realized that his telling of the paleo diet was a close match to where I already was. Today, I'm only running half as much, eating a little more, and drinking more frequently, but the soft drinks and most packaged foods are gone without regret. I've gained a little back, but I'm still wearing the same medium size clothes two years later. It took an overall lifestyle shift, but it had a successful and sustainable result.

PATRICIA CASHION

AUSTIN, TEXAS

www.instinctcatering.com , www.shootforhealthy.com

I am always thrilled to share my results and my Paleo lifestyle. I started out in life pretty lean being a gymnast. I was always involved in sports and athletics when I was young. I was no stranger to the benefits of exercise. I was, however, a stranger to the best nutrition for my body. I started gaining weight during puberty, and then went up and down from there. Starting in 1988, I gained around 40 pounds in my first two years of college, from 130-135 to 170. It was awful! I felt disgusted! I couldn't believe that I had let late night pizza parties and class on the run ruin my body. I began to eliminate fast food and any snacks that I could not just eat ONE of: chips, snacks, pizza, most bread, and dairy. Although I knew that I was eating less of the bad stuff with these tweaks, my nutrition was still lacking on all levels. This elimination definitely helped, but it still wasn't enough!

Between the ages of 17-38 (1988-2008), the "yo-yo dieting" began; I would lose weight in the fall and gain it in the spring/summer. My weight was up and down before I knew it and it wasn't because I was working on it. It just happened. Some of the health issues that occurred during these years included an ACL right knee repair, menstrual issues, heart palpitations during pregnancy, decreased immunity, a stillbirth (first child), and a miscarriage (second child). In 2007, after three pregnancies, I had my first son. I was blessed to have no complications with him even though I wasn't doing anything different. I went from 148 pounds (size 8/10) to 196 pounds (size 14/16). :(

One day in April 2008, I was exercising pretty heavily. I went home and after a couple of hours nearly fainted. I thought maybe I just worked out too hard, but my heart was beating so hard that I went to the hospital. The doctor told me I may have the onset of diabetes. I told him he was crazy…heck, I didn't really even know what diabetes was. Something was going on inside of me, something I couldn't see…and it wasn't good! It worried me but I still did nothing for about another four or five months.

This is about the time when I saw a friend of mine who looked incredibly fit and healthy. I asked what she was doing to get such amazing results. She explained to me that she was a crossfitter and it was her cross fit program's synthesis of nutrition fused with a great exercise program - she ate paleo. Paleo…I had never heard of paleo.

I was so interested that I began my research on "paleo." The statistics backing this lifestyle of foods were completely logical. It just made sense! What I didn't understand was: WHY wasn't everyone eating these foods? Why did they live with diseases they did not have to? Still these questions go through my mind. The "Food Pyramid" just looked worse and worse. I jumped in and started Paleo right away. I was going to be healthy, and I immediately knew this was the way to do it, *from the inside out*. I was right!

I am always reading and researching Paleo. When I started Paleo in late 2008, I was about 70%

paleo. I followed Dr. Loren Cordain's first edition of *The Paleo Diet*. As the months went on, more and more information was surfacing on the internet and in book stores, allowing more in-depth, ongoing research. There is a world of great information on the subject. I would encourage everyone to please take the time to see how it can change your life.

I also kept hearing "healthy food doesn't taste good." How could we make it better so that people would make a conscious choice to create healthier nutritional habits? I decided to go back to school at Le Cordon Bleu College of Culinary Arts, in Austin Texas to learn the chemistry behind mixing and preparing food within paleo guidelines. I wanted to be able to create fine, palatable cuisine that met the specific health goals of those eating the Paleo way and to introduce my cuisine to all those who have not heard of paleo. I also kept hearing that having a week with a six to seven pound weight loss was not healthy. Really, if all you are consuming is healthy food, how can your body's own elimination of fat storage be bad? We have always heard that one to two pounds a week is healthy. I guess it is - if you are not eating healthy.

I immediately started seeing changes in my weight, inch loss, better overall body tone, energy level, and feeling healthier. This is when I started strict paleo. I SEE and FEEL the results today. My passion for paleo grew, and I was immersing myself in learning everything I could. I have been blessed to be in touch with some amazing paleo people. I have such a strong passion for sharing paleo with everyone and these connections make that all possible.

I have had opposition from a lot of people along the way. Some family members joined me and some didn't -for a little while - then they saw results, read about paleo, and it made logical sense to them. Eliminating grains, legumes, soy, sugar, dairy, vegetable oil, hydrogenated oil, and partially-hydrogenated oils can change your life!

I am thrilled with knowing that I have re-trained my body to crave the good foods, not the bad. I eat when I want, as much as I want, of healthy paleo foods. My body told me what was healthy and what was not, and if I cheated, I paid for it. Visualize that feeling of bloating after a nice meal at Olive Garden. That is NOT a normal feeling and it leaves you craving additional high-carb food an hour later. Eating Paleo does NOT leave you feeling that way. We eat a high protein, high fat diet, getting our carbs naturally through vegetables and fruits. When our bodies eat paleo, we end up feeling truly satisfied. No hunger pain, no food coma, and no bloating. I think that the protein intake is what keeps the body from craving.

I want to be healthy for my best friend and spouse, whom I wish to grow old with and that is why I am paleo. I want to be a fun, healthy mom for my five-year-old, providing him the best example and healthy lifestyle starting young. And I want to help others to eat foods that heal their bodies through proper nutrition.

The biggest benefit to me has been weight loss, body tone, conversion of fat to muscle, energy, and no additional heart issues. Not only did my body improve, but my mind is more alert and positive. I feel great! I no longer take ADHD medication or any other medication.

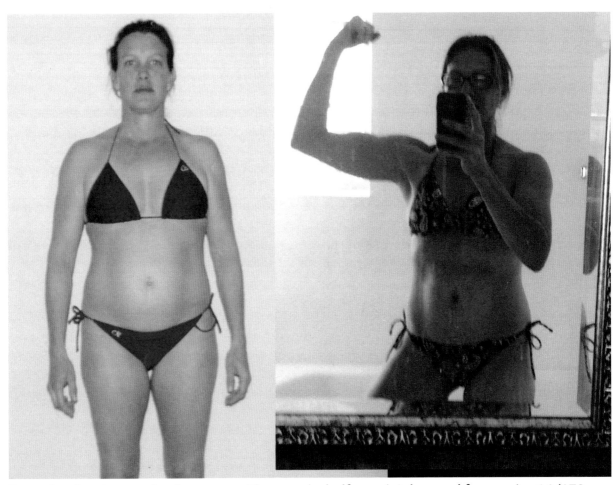

From the time I started paleo to now (three and a half years), I dropped from a size 14 (170 pounds) to a size 4 (124 pounds). I have maintained my size four a little less than three years now. Being able to maintain my current weight and size is awesome. I know that my body will continue to heal, from the inside out. I had too many years of improper nutrition, listening to next latest fad diet, and never knowing that what we were being told about nutrition was all backwards. There is information overload on what actually is healthy to eat. I can honestly say I believe paleo is the only way.

The first photo below was taken after being paleo for six months. In the second photo, I have maintained a size 4 for three and a half years now!

I am now officially a Paleo Chef! I only cook paleo foods. With my love for cooking paleo, in September 2012 I was fired up to build *Shoot for Healthy*, a food delivery company servicing Austin, Texas and the surrounding areas. We are already looking into branching out nationwide at a later date. I am also honored to partner with Michelle Norris to have created *INSTINCT Catering & Events, LLC*. This has been an amazing journey, and both businesses are about to launch as of this writing. We hope to reach as many people as we can.

Paleo IS my life. I live and breathe it. I am a whole-hearted Paleo Chef!

JENICE JOHNSON

DALLAS, TEXAS

www.jenicejohnson.com

I had no idea why I felt like I couldn't get out of bed in the mornings. I blamed it on depression. It was like the weight of the world was on me — I just felt so lethargic and worn out every morning. Like many people in America who may not know it, I have Hashimoto's Thyroiditis. It is an autoimmune disease that takes you through ups and downs of hypothyroidism and hyperthyroidism. I was diagnosed in 2008 when I was 30 years old.

I started taking Synthroid synthetic thyroid hormone and an additional medication called Cytomel that kick starts your thyroid. It seemed I felt good for a little while - but I hadn't changed my diet. The problem is that I was a sugar addict — big time. Because of a busy schedule, I often ate fast food at lunch or dinner swallowed down by a sugary slushy drink. Overall, I felt I ate decent (protein and veggies) but I would always fall into the habit of eating things like frosted sugar cookies. Sometimes they were my breakfast washed down with orange juice if I didn't get a breakfast taco in the morning from Sonic. Breads and very high-carb meals were a standard.

My weight went up to 204 pounds. Even after taking the medication and working out about three times a week, I was in the 190 range. Some of my old symptoms had come back too — feeling lethargic in the mornings and bouts of depression. I got really tired of constantly changing the levels of my medication. I started Jenny Craig and ate those horrible meals that still let you indulge regularly on pastry desserts. My weight never budged under 194 – and the food was expensive.

In 2010, I started a new job working for Native American Natural Foods — a company based on the Pine Ridge Indian Reservation that produces a natural bison protein bar called Tanka Bar. I noticed right away that we had a big following in the paleo community, and the product was even featured on Mark Sisson's site, marksdailyapple.com. All of the paleo success stories I began to hear helped me decide to give paleo a try…. this was right before holidays. What was I thinking?!?

I began to read Mark Sisson's *The Primal Blueprint* and was convinced that the potential health benefits were worth trying paleo.

Dropping bread and sugar was hands down the hardest part — especially at Christmas. I allowed myself a few cheats, but overall I stuck to my plan and lost about five pounds immediately. I didn't really commit to being 90% paleo until February 2011. My energy levels were significantly better. I got up easier in the mornings, and my mood had changed for the better. I FINALLY saw the number on the scale drop under 190, and I saw my clothes fit better.

Friends and family would ask me what I was doing differently. When I told them, they scoffed at the idea of dropping bread. For the most part everyone was supportive of the idea because I was looking and feeling better – but not without saying the usual, "I can't NOT eat bread" or "Your diet seems too high-maintenance."

A few people said that paleo seemed like a fad diet. I'll admit when I first started this journey, I didn't think I would keep it going as a lifestyle. However when I began to realize and understand how food was damaging my body, I knew this was about preserving my life and improving my health – permanently. I started going to a paleo-friendly doctor in 2011 and that is when it all came together for me. So much of how I used to eat ruined my gut – which I learned was directly connected to my immune system – and I have an autoimmune condition. It's pretty simple really – but none of my prior doctors knew anything about it and preferred to prescribe medication for me.

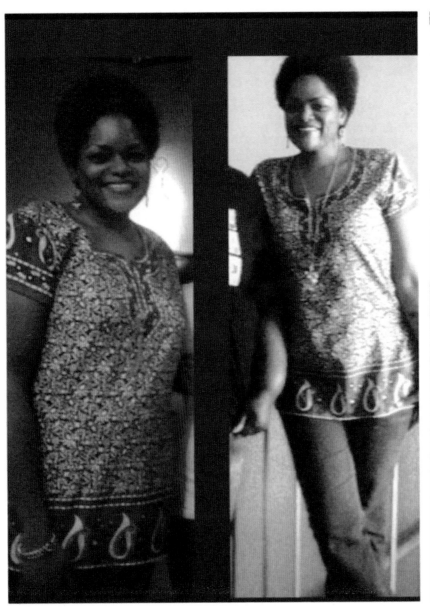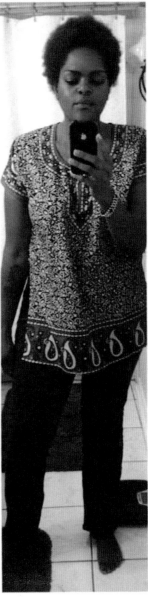

Through diet and proper supplementation to repair past damage, my blood work improved so much this year that my doctor told me that I could drop my thyroid medication if I wanted to. I was nervous about this because it seems that everyone in the medical field will tell you how much you need this medication - but they rarely, if ever, talk about diet. They don't tell you that regularly eating gluten can cause you a negative reaction. I see this still as a journey, and so far I've felt great without my meds.

Right now I stay consistently at 85-90% paleo. I will not pretend to say it has been easy 24/7, but to me it's a no-brainer — either you want to feel healthy and vibrant, or you don't. And when there are those days that I don't eat the best, I can REALLY feel the impact on my body.

It's like I am back in touch with myself. And it's pretty fascinating to see how differently my tastes have changed. Things that taste sweet are now way too sweet, and gluten may as well be a cannonball hitting my stomach. I also didn't know anything about fermented foods and now I swear by them and brew my own kombucha — something I would have never tried doing before.

Because of the years of damage to my body, I still take supplements. But I no longer take any prescriptions. I regularly take a fermented fish oil, vitamin D, and Oxicell, a glutathione cream. I still work out about three times a week, but every day I at least try to stay active with something for at least 20 minutes (whether lifting, squats, or walking). I find my biggest challenge with a crazy schedule is making time to have a full workout more regularly. One thing you learn on this path is that you make time for what is important to you. That said, now at 34, I weigh 184 — 20 pounds lighter than when I was in my late 20s.

I know I still have more room to improve, but the road doesn't feel as daunting as it did years ago. I enjoy having energy – and feeling more in tune with my body. That has been my favorite part about this journey — being more aware of how my body reacts to certain foods instead of just assuming bad reactions are "normal" because we are conditioned that certain negative nuances in how our body responds to certain foods is "normal" and should be fixed with prescription medicine rather than food.

What is fantastic is what paleo does for your mind. You begin to believe that things are possible instead of just thinking those are lofty words you see on colorful Facebook memes. You see where you started, and appreciate where you are headed. Your confidence to obtain your dreams becomes more prominent in your life. It's all part of the lifestyle. The improvements are not just on your body – but your mind, emotions, and spirit.

PATTY

RENO, NEVADA

My name is Patty and I'm a 47 year old whole foods health addict. I've never been overly fat; to the contrary, I've been skinny-fat for most of my life. For years I've been on a quest to find out what we, as humans, were "designed" to eat, what types of foods my body performs best on, and what the best form of exercise is for optimal health. Because I don't have any severe food intolerances or allergies, my path on this quest has been quite varied.

I grew up on a small farm in Wisconsin where we raised a steer, a pig, had chickens, and grew most of our own vegetables. I also had wheat, cereals, pies, cakes, soda, and most other SAD (Standard American Diet) items that most people have had. I watched my Mother take teaspoons of cod liver oil, eat liver, and other supplements to aid her in her own personal voyage for optimal health. I think seeing her do this, coupled with the environment I was raised in, engrained in me a strong value for taking care of myself.

I think my first round of eating style was the low-fat, whole-wheat craze. Being female, I was searching for that perfect fitness model figure, and I would do just about anything to get that toned body 'they" said I'd get if I followed this eating program. My heaviest weight was close to 160 pounds. At 5'7", and pretty proportionate, I managed to hide my weight pretty well and I never appeared overweight by most peoples' standards. But for me, the extra weight I was carrying was unacceptable. I stuffed as many non-fat foods down my gullet that I could find. Of course, everything fit neatly into a wrapper or container, and had an expiration date printed on it with an ingredient list a mile long which I couldn't pronounce. I had no clue what most of the ingredients were. But the literature, TV commercials, and government gurus said it was what I needed to eat to make me healthy.

The thing that stands out most in my mind was the gas I had from switching over to so much whole wheat - and the fact that my period stopped - from what I now think was too little dietary fat. I ate this way for many years. I was also a gym rat and was under the impression that I had to do endless hours of high intensity cardio training to keep the fat from attaching itself to various parts of my female physique. I had lost a little weight, hovering around 150 most of the time but the stubborn fat still remained.

Next up was the vegetarian route - I ate oodles and oodles of fruit and vegetables, lots of rice, quinoa, and noodles - no poultry or meat with the exception of occasional sushi nights with my husband. After reading lots of vegetarian blogs, I decided that I should be doing a raw vegan diet. That would give me perfect health! Or so I thought. So I did it, for a summer. I ate a lot of salad, drank a lot of smoothies, and sought up creative ways to eat all of my foodstuffs in their raw state. My choices were very limited, nothing was ever cooked, and I think if I had stayed on it for any real length of time other than the three or four months of summer, I probably would've developed some health issues. I remember that I was always cold that summer.

After stopping the raw vegan diet, I returned to a mostly vegetarian way of life which I did for several years. The fat still remained and even though I was eating "healthy", my stomach protruded like I was four months pregnant.

Following my years of vegetarian/vegan/raw vegan eating experimentation, I returned to what is viewed as the normal way of eating. I went back to low or non-fat, and whole wheat. Back to tracking caloric intake, and worrying about fat content. Back to the world of no avocados, butter, or whole eggs. Back to killing myself in the gym doing endless hours of cardio. After all of this, I plateaued at 147 pounds on a 5'7" frame.

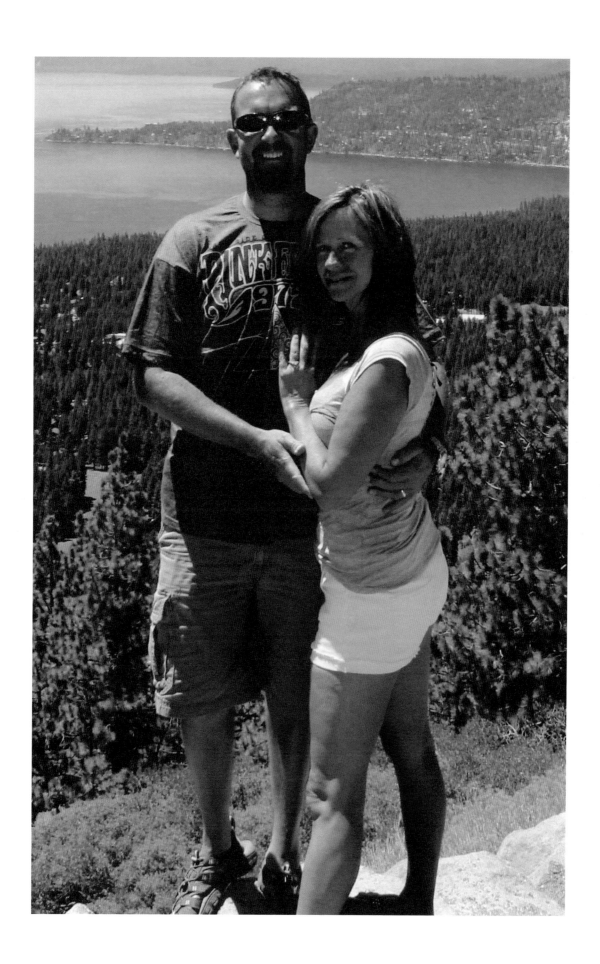

During this timeframe I was introduced to Beachbody and the P90X workouts, which led me to the online forums, which led me to a man who talked about being able to eat all the fat and red meat he wanted. He boasted about laying on the couch and the fat just melting off his body. He led me to a website hosted by Mark Sisson from which I was introduced to the book titled The Primal Blueprint. I downloaded the book to my Kindle and immediately began reading it. The principles seemed to make sense so I decided to give the eating plan a try. That was in February of 2011.

Through my research and love affair with Google I came upon the many paleo websites and found a wonderful forum filled with educated, like minded people that accepted my paleo eating patterns. Fortunately my transition to this way of life hasn't produced too many obstacles. My family and friends are supportive and quite frankly, they are just used to me trying different things and changing my eating ways. To be perfectly honest I really wouldn't care if they weren't cheering me on. This is my health and my life, not theirs.

I think the hardest part of going paleo was the re-wiring of my brain. Being bombarded with all the "whole wheat is a dietary must and eggs raise your cholesterol" mumbo jumbo over the decades is hard to forget. I just keep in daily contact with my friends on my forum and they help me to re-focus when I need to, and I continue to research and read on my own so I'm not stuck in a non-progressive bubble. I have routine blood work done to track my numbers and everything is spot on. My workouts have morphed to more of a weight training instead of chronic cardio approach, focusing on building strength instead of burning calories. I'm only in the gym 3 times a week for about 45 minutes per session and my stair master has been replaced by a good paced walk. I also concentrate on meditation and getting adequate amounts of sleep each night as these are also important components of the lifestyle.

People ask me what my favorite part about living this way is and there are many, but I guess it's the freedom. The freedom to eat all the real food I want. The freedom to not worry about dietary fat making me fat. The freedom from mimicking a hamster on a wheel; running and running and getting nowhere.

The changes in my body composition aren't drastic, but they are significant. Right now I'm sitting at 135 pounds with more muscle than I've ever had and I feel absolutely fantastic. I really do love this way of life and I'm excited to see the upcoming changes in my spirit and in my body as the years progress. I also hope to be an inspiration to those around me as they watch me transform almost effortlessly and dispel all the myths that we've been told for many years.

RACHEL FLOWERS

DALLAS, TEXAS

r_c_flowers@yahoo.com , alternefit.wordpress.com

Several years ago, I began a quest. It started when I lost some weight and wanted to make sure I kept it off. At the same time, I got interested in health and wellness. At the time, I was a

"Pollo-Vegetarian" - meaning I was eating chicken and some fish, but not red meat. For the 13 years before that, I was a full-fledged Vegetarian, and even tried Veganism for 2 months. I was also very unhealthy. I was at first overweight at 5', 2" and 140 pounds, and then underweight at 97 pounds. My health conditions were pretty severe. I was diagnosed with bi-polar disorder, and a psychiatrist wanted to put me on experimental anti-seizure medication for treatment. I refused. Also, my immune system was weak. Every year, 4 times a year, for most of my life, I got extremely severe strep throat that was antibiotic-resistant and gave me fevers so high that I would temporarily go color blind. I had hay fever and felt tired all the time. My gums were receding and I lost two teeth. As you can see, I was not well.

For my bi-polar disorder, I went to a homeopath/herbalist. He prescribed me a tincture tailored specifically to me and something called "a blue tube of homeopathic medicine." This did help, but it did not keep me stable all of the time. When I got strep throat, I would go to the emergency room. It was always a difficult trek. I would have to take an antibiotic injection as well as start a prescription of antibiotics. The injection, which was supposed to begin 'working' within 24 hours, never worked well for me at all.

When my allergies kicked in hard, I suffered. No form of allergy medication worked! My eyes constantly watered and I was often heard to say "I feel like I'm under water!" I even begged an allergist to give me allergy shots, to no avail. Apparently, the allergists I went to did not give allergy shots unless the person registered as asthmatic on the breath test. I passed, albeit barely, and so I did not qualify.

The final problem was with my weight. I was very heavy. Once I finally began to lose weight, I also started looking into ways to keep the weight off and be healthy at the same time. I must say, I was not wise about health back then. I thought I could keep the weight off by just limiting my calories to 500-900 a day and taking some 'carb blockers.' I also joined the YMCA and did the elliptical machine for at least an hour. I signed up for all sorts of workout classes as well (swimmercise, crunch class, treadmill classes, and even running). All of these things did work for weight loss. In fact, it worked too well. I got down to a measly 97 pounds. At 5', 2", I was way too thin! I was also still miserable with allergies, lethargy, tooth and gum problems, mood swings, and the never-ending strep throat. There had to be something I could do!

Right around the time I began losing weight, I met the man who is now my husband. We casually dated for a while, and realized we were falling for each other. I found out that he was a diabetic (Type II). He was getting a divorce from his ex, and losing his insurance. That worried me. How would he take care of himself and get his medications without insurance? There had to be another way. How did people with diabetes take care of themselves in the past, when insulin was not available?

With this in my mind, and with my own health problems still plaguing me, I began to research. I went online and read everything I could find on diabetes. I sought out podcasts and radio shows about health. That was when I found a podcast called 'Underground Wellness' by Sean Croxton. It literally had everything I was looking for! I listened intently to all of the available shows. I took notes. I followed links from the show notes. What was being said on this

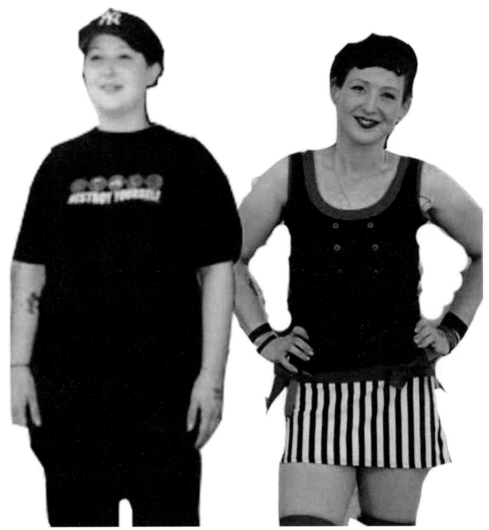

podcast made complete sense to me - it was logical, based in science and history, and gave me hope. I decided at that point, "Yes, I think I'm going to actually eat meat again; not just chicken and fish, but red meat too!"

Of course I was very nervous. I hadn't eaten red meat in 13 years! How would my body react to it? I didn't want to take a chance with store-bought meat. If I was going to do this, I was going to do it in the healthiest way I thought I could. I went out and bought a quarter pound of grass fed ground beef. I told the guy at the meat counter that I had not eaten meat in 13 years, and would like to know if he had suggestions for cooking and eating it. He said I might just try to eat it IN something, like a casserole or a pizza. When I got home with my grass fed beef, I searched for recipes for 'Low-Carb and Paleo pizza,' and I found one! It used a cauliflower crust, and did contain cheese. I thought, "Well….let's do this!" I followed the recipe to a T, and prepared to take the plunge into being truly healthy via my grass fed meat! You might have heard that some people who are vegetarians for a long time and begin to eat meat again get sick the first time they try. I was worried about this, but it was all for naught. I did not get sick. I did not feel bad in any way. Because the cauliflower pizza went well, I decided it was definitely time to up the ante. I went back and bought more ground beef. Then I bought a steak. Then I bought another steak. Sure enough, I started noticing a change.

Now, instead of eating processed soy garbage like soy hot dogs, tofu burgers, seitan, and textured vegetable protein, I eat REAL foods like grass fed beef, fatty fish, steaks, liver, and much more! Instead of carbing up on breads, pastas, chips, crackers, and white potatoes, I lavish my tummy with a variety of vegetables, sweet potatoes, beef jerky, and macadamia nuts. I cook real meals instead of microwaving boxed garbage. My palate has become what I like to consider 'a foodie palate.'

Today, at 115 pounds, I do not suffer from mood swings. My allergies, while still around, are greatly reduced. I have not gotten strep throat in 2 years, and haven't even gotten sick. My cavities and gum disease have come to a halt. I now have energy that not only helps me get through the day, but also assists me in gaining strength for my weight lifting and crossfit days! I feel rested and well. Don't get me wrong - these changes did not occur over night. It took several months before I noticed a change in energy and mood. It took even longer to realize that I wasn't getting sick. And now it has been two years, and I am happy with my 115 pound weight. My allergies are much less challenging these days- although there is still room for improvement. Overall, it has been 2 years of constant change and realization of health! I do not go to doctors these days. I take no prescriptions or medications. My PMS, which was getting pretty bad, is lightening up now. I am starting to see better hair growth and improvement in sleep. These are all positive signs that what I am doing is helping me inside and out!

My mom gets it. She follows my advice and has taken her own steps. She will still occasionally eat corn chips or something like that; however, she does try very hard stay away from grains, legumes, and seed oils most of the time. I have also been a positive influence on friends and co-workers, many who have removed grains and tried to stay away from most processed foods. They ask me questions and continue to stay positive in their own lives as well. People around me do see the results, and they want in! And I am more than willing to help! After all, one step at a time turns into a great lifestyle change. This is not just a diet. It is a way of living that I believe we should all be familiar with and strive toward. It is in our genes and our history.

Committing to the change feels good! Amazing things really can happen! It goes far beyond weight loss! I mean, the fact that my bi-polar disorder is null and void now, with no medication, has got to show that! The commitment to lifestyle change is well worth the rewards!

HEIDI M.

BOZEMAN, MONTANA

After a bout with severe exhaustion and two pregnancies that were very hard on my body, I found myself about 100 pounds overweight and feeling unhealthy on a daily basis. I did not have any specific medical conditions, but I was suffering the effects of being overweight: fatigue, joint pain, headaches, and general malaise. I wasn't really exercising - other than being a stay-at-home mom of two kids under the age of 3. I was eating what I thought then was a healthy diet: Low fat, whole grains, and counting calories. I had even signed up for an online group to help me track my food and count calories so I could 'eat for weight loss.' I was not successful with weight loss by just changing my diet, so I decided to add some focused exercise to my routine.

About 1.5 months before I began to eat paleo, at the age of 38, I started doing some light exercise at home 4-5 days per week. Yoga and Wii Fitness games mostly, with walking mixed in. A few pounds came off, but not what I was expecting. Then a friend told me about a challenge she was doing at her crossfit gym. It was a Whole30 challenge (a specific protocol of the paleo diet www.whole30.com), followed by 60 days of paleo eating. She had amazing results with her Whole30, so I decided to do some research and set a start date for my own Whole30. I planned, shopped, and prepped for this 30-day challenge and was more than impressed with (a) how I felt better almost immediately (b) how effortless my weight loss became, and c) HOW EASY IT ALL WAS. Heck, all I did was change the kind of food I ate. I wasn't stressing out about counting calories every time I felt hungry. I simply ate whenever I felt like it and kept the right ingredients on hand. In the first month, I effortlessly lost 10 pounds.

I completed my first Whole30 and I felt so great that I turned around and started another one right away – and lost another 10 pounds. When I started, I honestly thought it would be just a 30-day challenge and then on to the next plan. Looking back, it was a no-brainer to see that food really does make a difference. After that I continued to eat paleo with a more strict Whole30 tossed in here and there when I felt I was starting to slide or my weight loss seemed to slow down. I have been paleo for just over a year and a half now and I am loving it. Eating real, whole foods is the easy part. I think the hardest part has been explaining to other people why I have decided to eat this way.

During this time I also gradually started increasing the intensity of my exercise. I started a running program after my second month and by the 6 month mark, I was going to my first crossfit class. I went to crossfit for a month and then went on to do a round of P90X, a round of Insanity, and have continued to do home workouts intermixed with walking and hiking. The hardest part of trying to keep a good fitness routine is definitely my crazy schedule. I have learned to maximize my parenting time and have managed to successfully integrate working out and taking care of the children.

I did not intend to "completely change my life," but lo and behold, my life has changed. At 40, after more than a year and a half of eating paleo and exercising regularly, I am no longer

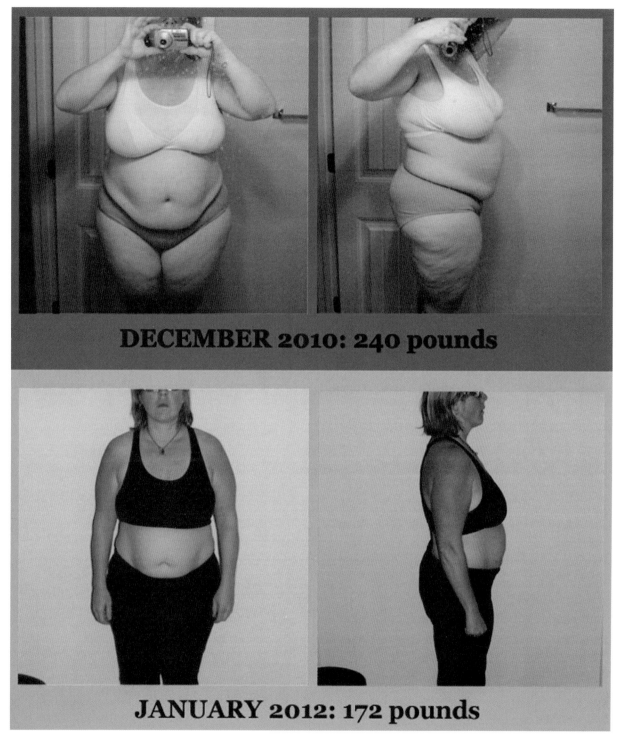

DECEMBER 2010: 240 pounds

JANUARY 2012: 172 pounds

suffering the effects of being severely overweight. The fatigue, joint pain, headaches, and general malaise have subsided.

My menstrual cycles are now regular – they had never before been regular without taking birth control medication. My skin is clear all month long too. I have lost nearly 70 pounds. I can keep up with my kids and my husband again. I enjoy playing outside again, and I really feel like ME again after all these years!

TIFFANY

NEW FAIRFIELD, CONNECTICUT

I discovered the paleo lifestyle through my mother in the late fall of 2011. She struggled with her health for many years and when she started I certainly did not buy into it. I am a Junior and a mid and long distance runner with almost 4 years of training and competition at state, regional, and national events. I train rigorously 6 days a week and I take my diet very seriously. How could I possibly NOT fuel my body with pasta? I need carbohydrates to perform! Paleo seemed to go against everything I was taught!

I noticed positive results in my mother's health and her physical improvements. She had more energy, more stamina, and generally more LIFE. She was happier, calmer, and younger looking. My father slowly converted this past winter and I saw some positive changes in him as well. He dropped weight, put on muscle very quickly, and was able to manage his cholesterol without medication. By mid spring of 2012 we were all following a paleo meal plan. I rebelled and insisted they keep bread in the freezer and prepare pasta for me pre-competition.

I had become a vegetarian for several months as a result of watching Food, Inc. at school. The unethical treatment of animals disturbed me and I found myself unable to look at meat. I did not fare as well in competition and for the first time in my life, gained weight. Knowing what I had learned from my mother about paleo and how the lifestyle focused on sustainable farming and the ethical treatment of animals, I started to reconsider my options.

One evening before a race, I came to dinner and did not see pasta and meat sauce with a side of spinach. I was mortified! My mother knew my routine! How could she do this to me?

Instead, she had a carrot ginger soup with coconut milk, roasted sweet potatoes and beef patties with sautéed vegetables. She had with her a spreadsheet listing all the nutritional values that were in my meal and compared it with what was in my typical pre-race menu. I am a science geared student with a goal to get into medicine. The numbers were there, and I knew she had a point. What I didn't know was how my body would respond.

I ran a great race the following day. I was now willing to give paleo a serious go. My mother researched to build meal plans around my competition schedule. I was convinced I needed to carb-load before a race so we developed meals with nutrient dense squashes, pumpkins, sweet potatoes and fruits. Nuts and unsweetened dried fruits became a staple at home. I occasionally consumed full-fat yogurt, milk, and cheeses. We started to track macronutrients and discovered that every meal she prepared was at the very least equivalent in total carbohydrates to my typical pasta dish but with a HUGE vitamin/mineral kick that grains did not provide.

I noticed that my eczema and skin irritations, including facial break-outs were much more under control. I would occasionally indulge in bread and wheat treats and noticed my eczema flare up again intensely. If this was happening externally, what on earth could be

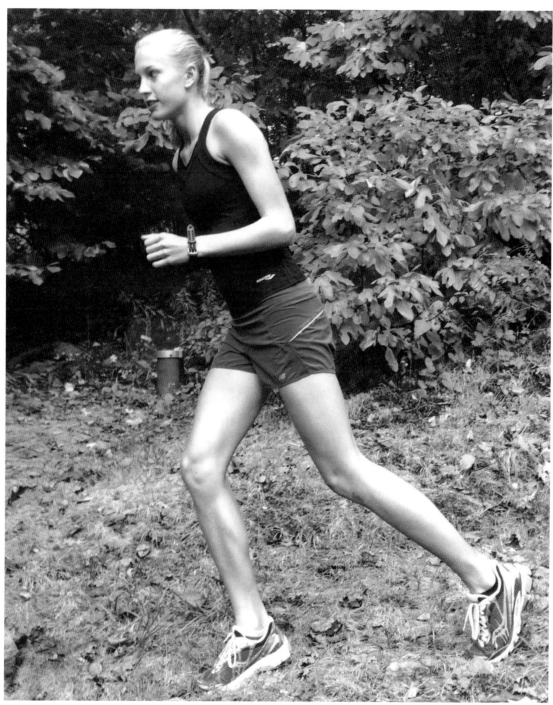

going on inside my body? I was convinced to give up grains entirely. My diet now consists of grass-fed meats, eggs from pasture-raised hens, wild caught fish, vegetables, fruits, coconut milk, coconut and olive oil, nuts, seeds, and some raw dairy. We even bake some awesomely delicious treats using coconut flour. I have never felt like I was missing out on anything.

As far as my medical issues are concerned, I had a lifelong issue with eczema, chronic bronchitis, asthma and severe seasonal allergies. Though I overcame the upper respiratory issues earlier, I still struggled with eczema and allergies.

At the start of my Paleo journey, I was just under 5', 8" and weighed 135 pounds. I am now 5', 8" and 122 pounds. Weight loss was never my goal, but I have noticed my stomach flatten and more muscle mass in my abdomen and arms, not just my legs. My body has definitely improved its ability to build muscle. My moods have stabilized and my menstrual cycle has normalized. My eczema is completely gone, my allergies are no longer a concern, and my stamina has improved. I notice I heal faster, recover quicker, and my overall clarity of thinking has changed.

What has been the most striking change after adopting a paleo lifestyle has been my mindset. I feel a major shift in confidence. I feel that following a paleo template gives me a competitive edge, because I know when I step on that starting line and I see the rows of hundreds of athletes before me, not one of them is fueling their Ferrari with jet fuel. And this knowledge gives me confidence for my race. When I feel great, I run great.

I have also witnessed an improvement on my performance. I have PRed in each of my competitive events. My first PR was exhilarating, but I wasn't quick to attribute it to my lifestyle change. But the second, third and every subsequent PR truly made be a believer!

My greatest challenge has been explaining to my teammates why I eat the way I do. It is difficult to explain why grains are harmful when people look at you in disbelief, or throw some stupid commentary from something they heard or read. It is especially difficult to attend my Foods class and have to forego the bread or pasta dishes they make. But I do!

I know my own personal experiment is a testimony to the effectiveness of the paleo lifestyle. Every win. Every PR. Every time I wake up and can breathe well or don't have to reach for hydrocortisone has contributed to my firm belief that I am Paleo For Life.

ADRIENNE JESS

LAS VEGAS, NEVADA

All my life I have struggled with my weight and the foods that I eat. Since I was a child – beginning around the age of eight – I would often have to take antacids to fight the chronic heartburn I suffered. My parents assumed that I had digestive issues similar to that of my Grandpa and didn't think anything of it. Not that they didn't care that I was suffering, but I wasn't standing there complaining about it – so it went largely untreated. They also thought that I was simply a picky eater. The reality was that the foods that I avoided made me sick to my stomach.

When I became a teenager, I was "upgraded" to the longer-acting acid suppressants. I was a short girl, and even though I was very active – hiking, biking, riding horses since I was four – I never could lose weight. I was probably 5', 1" and 140 pounds when I finished high school. Then I discovered beer and college parties, and was up to 160 pounds at one point – and I eventually grew to 5', 5".

Years went by and the heartburn was almost constant. I did lose some weight, but it was the result of working as a professional in the horse business. I was pulling 12-14 hour days (or longer) and working 6-7 days per week. Despite being naturally high energy most of my life, I started to feel sluggish and tired. I developed gastro-esophageal reflux disease (GERD) and had trouble keeping foods down. Everything came back up, which made eating a real adventure. I tried avoiding spicy foods, onions, tomatoes… all the things that seemed to bother other members of my family – with no success.

I also always seemed to be injuring something: I developed tendonitis, my back ached, my hands hurt, and I had stress fractures in both wrists.

In 2009, I developed a near insatiable craving for heavy wheat beers. Every day for a week my boyfriend (now husband) would take me to my favorite local restaurant and I would drink 2-3 pints of beer. My stomach stated to feel like a stone in my gut. I started to feel constantly rolling waves of nausea. I was miserable. I went to my chiropractor's office for acupuncture, and this helped me lose some of my gut again.

A naturopath at the local clinic suggested trying a specific carbohydrate diet – and I began putting two and two together and realized that I was practically living exclusively off of bread, pasta, and other types of wheat-based items. The gluten-free trend was just starting, and people were realizing that not everyone who had sensitivity to gluten was a Celiac. And it was then when I decided to completely rid my diet of all things gluten. So began my days of reading labels, inquiring about ingredients at restaurants, and all the little things that you must do when you make a serious change to your eating.

Some things didn't really change though. I simply swapped gluten-filled items with gluten-free items. I changed the habit but not the behavior. I was like an alcoholic who opted for O'Doul's beer instead of Widmer.

I began feeling even more weak and tired. At the time I was working 40 hours per week in an office and was also working 30 hours with my horses, trying to get my training and lesson business off the ground. I was struggling at both my jobs. I would be so exhausted I would just lie down and cry. My blood sugar was going crazy. I have suffered from hypoglycemia all my life, but it was getting more severe. I *had* to eat something at night before I went to bed – especially if we had gone out for a couple of drinks – otherwise I would wake up so "low" that I couldn't physically get out of bed. My husband had to carry me to bed or to the couch on a number of occasions. I would get severe head rushes and would almost pass out.

In December of 2010 I contacted a friend's naturopath and had her draw blood and run tests. It was determined that I was severely anemic. She also checked my thyroid, but thankfully all was well. She suggested I try the blood type diet, which for my type meant no meats except chicken or turkey, some fish (which I don't like), little to no dairy, only soy products, etc. I was to be getting all my iron from beans, vegetables, and iron supplements; in theory we would heal my gut with probiotics.

I wasn't feeling any better on the blood type diet despite following it to a T. I was getting even more frustrated with how I felt, the lack of weight loss (I was around 145 at this time), the

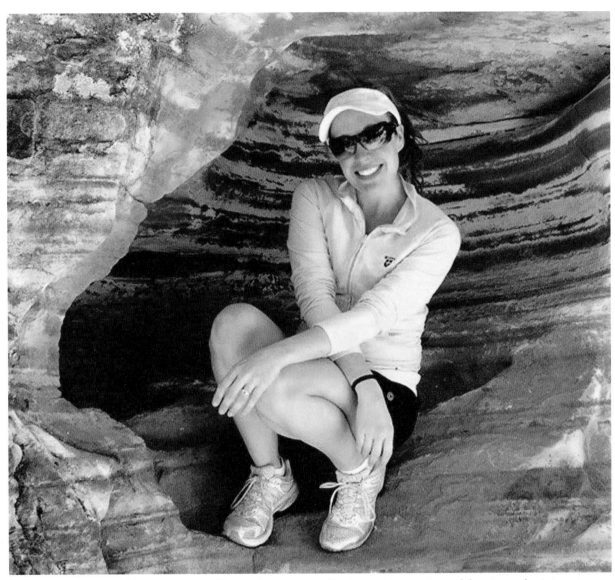

lack of energy, and just my overall physical state of being. I was miserable at work. I was too tired to ride my horses or keep trying to grow my business. My health took a toll on my life. I began seeing posts about paleo on Facebook from a good friend of mine. I began reading the things she was posting and began studying it. My chiropractor then brought it up during one adjustment and I grilled her for more information. I began slowly changing things in my diet toward a paleo plan. I had noticed that beans gave me heartburn, and so did the gluten-free bagels that I liked. I started eating more meat again.

By fall of 2011 I had completely switched to paleo. I immediately noticed the difference in my energy levels. I dropped down to 128 pounds and was easily able to make it through my long and physically taxing workdays. My joint pain improved dramatically, only surfacing in areas where I had severe injury – but even there not to the extremes it had in the past when I awoke feeling crippled at times.

love that I get to enjoy a steak at any time of the day, and I get to put butter on my broccoli.

People are always surprised by the amount of food I eat despite that I maintain my slim figure (130 pounds today). I work out every day (cardio and strength training), and I don't feel guilty on days I don't.

To this day the thing that surprises me the most is the energy level that I have. I am excited and happy all the time and I am just enjoying life so much more. My husband is completely supportive of this lifestyle and I am so blessed. He enjoys the meals I make and doesn't complain on our shopping trips. He truly is an incredible person! I am never leaving the Paleo lifestyle; it has made THE biggest difference for me. I just wish others would be more open-minded about trying it. I personally believe it is the best way for everyone to achieve optimum health.

JULES GOODMAN

SOUTHERN CALIFORNIA

http://is.gd/paleosocal

I just recently turned 34. I have been overweight since after having my youngest child almost 10 years ago. My highest weight was 169 pounds. I was used to being between 112 and 117 pounds. I never went over 117 pounds when I wasn't pregnant until after my fourth child was born. I felt like I had gained a whole other me, but I didn't care enough. I saw what was happening to my body but I had become depressed due to things out of my control. I developed Obsessive Compulsive Disorder (OCD) and General Anxiety Disorder. I lived this way for years. I hadn't had a clear head in a long time and I didn't think I ever would again. I had thought the brain fog was something I was going to have to learn to live with.

I used to eat salt and vinegar chips by the bag! And candy whenever I could get my hands on it. I drank at least 4 cans of soda a day! My diet and my family's diet was full of pasta, bread, white potatoes, and processed food. We also ate a lot of fast food. I was completely naive to what I was doing to my body and what was happening to my children's health. I knew we didn't eat healthy but I didn't know just how unhealthy we were eating.

Paleo came into my life when I learned I had a stomach infection called Helicobactor Pylori, or H. Pylori for short. I suspect I picked it up at a fast food joint that I went to with my youngest son. It's a bad bacteria that burrows into the mucous lining of the stomach and causes a lot of pain, stomach upset, and acid reflux. I had to take an antacid and two antibiotics to get rid of it. Once I finished my antibiotics I got another blood test that came back positive. After getting the second positive I researched how to get rid of my infection naturally.

I took natural supplements temporarily and changed my diet at the suggestion of a chiropractor I saw. I had still been experiencing the symptoms of H. Pylori and had even landed in the ER with sharp stomach pains that were never diagnosed. Paleo relieved my symptoms. It was so nice to eat something and not experience pain or stomach upset. I also noticed the changes in my outside appearance and my mental well being. I was starting to lose my stomach! My skin looked better! My OCD and anxiety symptoms started to lessen!

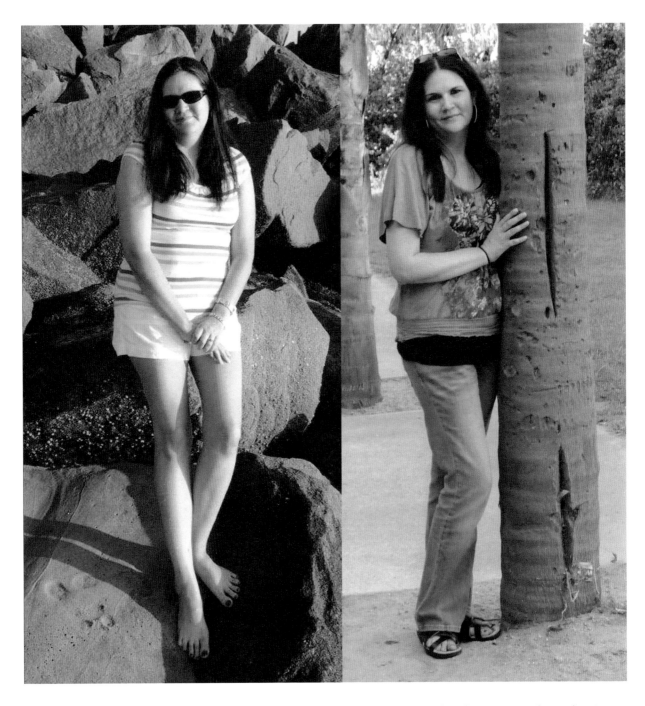

The brain fog I had been experiencing disappeared! I was relieved to be wrong about having to live the rest of my life with all these conditions, I realized I had found what I had been looking for.

That was when I realized how much food really matters. My moods improved and I started to regain some energy. Paleo helped me beat my addiction to soda. I had tried many times over the years to stop drinking it and failed. It helped to know that the bad things I was putting into my body would prevent me from getting rid of my infection. I wanted to get better! And I did!

I tested again for H. Pylori, and the result was negative! I almost cried. Hearing that diagnosis did not send me back to eating chips though! Although I am not entirely sure if it was my diet that cured the infection, the way I used to eat was not an option anymore.

I have learned so much in the last three months. I wish I knew years ago what I know now!

It wasn't an easy road though. When I first changed my diet to paleo, I experienced what is called the "carb flu." I was so weak and cranky. I didn't want to keep eating paleo and even contemplated quitting a few weeks in. But I didn't because of my infection. Without it, I may have never changed. It's said that nothing worth having comes easy and I believe that to be true.

Right now I'm trying to master my sugar cravings and it has been a struggle - but one I believe will be worth it in the end. Paleo hasn't just helped me. It has helped my family as well. My oldest son has been battling high triglycerides for years. He started gaining too much weight at 8 years old. Now he eats Paleo and goes to the gym regularly and the weight is melting off! He's gone from 235 pounds to 208 pounds in 3 months. My youngest son, who was also diagnosed with H. Pylori, is eating paleo to rid himself of the infection and we hope his next test leaves us as happy as mine did.

My husband, who had fought me tooth and nail on this diet, has now lost 43 pounds! Our oldest daughter transitioned with no complaints and is happy to eat healthy while our youngest daughter moans and groans a bit but for the most part she does ok.

I feel we have seen positive changes all around! I'm walking as much as I can and currently am working my way up to 5 miles every other day. I even got my husband to walk a mile with me once! I couldn't be happier since discovering the paleo lifestyle and I for one am never turning back!

MICHAEL KOVACS

PEMBERTON MEADOWS, BRITISH COLUMBIA, CANADA

Between the ages of 14-16 years, I was fairly athletic, stood 5', 7", weighed 130 pounds, and was lean and muscular. I was a member of my high school track and field club, on the volleyball team, and played badminton – but long distance running was my specialty. I had great stamina and could run a 6-minute mile without much effort. I competed provincially and made it to the finals. At age 14, I competed in the Columbia Valley Half Marathon and finished first in my age group.

At age 16, I started cycling and went on several long distance cycling trips, including a 230 km ride from Vancouver to Mt. Bake, and a 130 km ride from Vancouver to Harrison Hot Springs. Life was great, without a care in the world. At 17 years old, I moved out on my own. I got a job as a longshoreman after my uncle "dragged me by the ear" to the Vancouver docks to get registered. My uncle, grandfather, and great-grandfather had also worked the docks. It took several years to gradually move up the boards, but I eventually got more work. I gained considerable weight because much of the work was back breaking labor, and I ate like a horse. By the end of 1994, I was pushing 165 pounds. By 2 years later, I gained 20 more pounds, to 185 pounds. In 1995, became certified as a mobile equipment operator and from then I no longer did as much manual labor. I was now driving tractor trailers and forklifts. In 1998 I received more training as a Heavy Lift Truck Driver and Rubber Tired Gantry. At that time I tipping the scales at 220 pounds, getting sicker and sicker, catching a cold 2 or 3 times a year, and wound up with bronchial pneumonia a few times.

Family members would joke that I snored louder than a 747 – but it was no joke. It got so bad, I often found myself sleeping alone because my wife went to sleep on the coach or would demote me to the couch. One time we went on a road trip to visit family and shared a motel room with my sister-in-law and her two kids, the kids went to sleep in the car and my sister-in-law slept in the bathroom. The snoring didn't bother my wife all that much, but my sleep apnea sure did. My wife would give me a shot in the ribs with her elbow to get me to start breathing again. This happened quite often and was having a negative effect on my wife's health too, not just mine. But worse than the snoring and the sleep apnea was my acid reflux. The pain was so bad that I couldn't go anywhere without my antacids. I would chew them morning, noon, and night, 3 or 4 at a time. I couldn't go to sleep without propping myself up with pillows.

My doctor told me I needed to avoid foods containing cholesterol, red meat, watch my fat intake, and eat lots of healthy whole grains, fresh fruits, and vegetables. So I followed her advice for about 6 months, eating very little meat. The meat I did eat was mostly skinless boneless chicken breast and fish. I was eating lots of whole wheat pasta salads with low fat dressing, drinking soy milk, using soy margarine, and eating lots of fruit and vegetables. But my health continued to decline. By 2008 I was 240 pounds and diagnosed with asthma, pre-diabetes, and high blood pressure. My typical blood pressure reading was 160/95. I was put on steroid inhalers for the asthma, and told that I would be taking them for the rest of my life. My doctor suggested the asthma was caused by my work environment, and blamed the high blood pressure on my stress. She wanted to give me statins for my high cholesterol in addition to blood pressure meds. I refused and said I would like to find a more natural approach,

By July 2009 I was 260 pounds, my back ached from walking the shortest of distances. Climbing stairs became a chore, and my breathing was impaired. The time was perfect for my good friend and co-worker to encourage me to read *The Protein Power Lifeplan* by Drs. Michael and Mary Dan Eades.

The more I read, the more I could not put it down. I burned through that book in three days. I wasn't even finished reading this book yet and decided to empty my pantry and cupboards of everything with grains, sugar, starch, MSG. Things such as boxes of cereal, pasta, bags of bread, pretzels, beans, juice crystals, pop, anything that would cause my blood sugar to go up went into a garbage bag. I got a glucose monitor and watched my blood sugar carefully.

Within 2 weeks I was down 14 pounds, was able to throw away the antacids because my acid reflux stopped completely. By the end of the first month I was down 30 pounds, my snoring

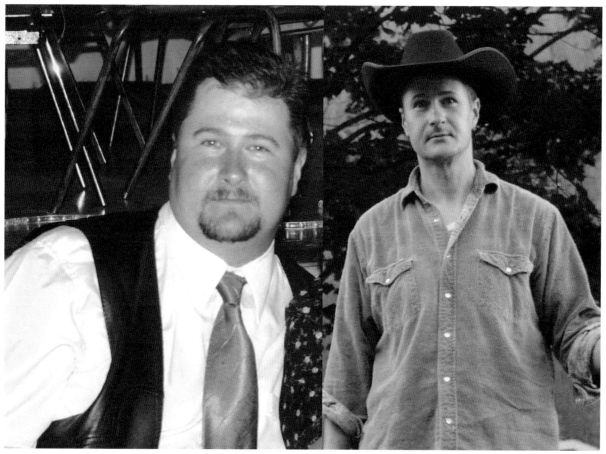

and sleep apnea came to an end. For the first time in years I was sleeping through the night and waking up well rested. I lost almost a pound a day every of the next month. Both my blood pressure and blood sugar dropped into normal range. My sinuses were clear as a bell and I hadn't had a need for my inhalers for over a month.

My last asthma attack was in September 2009 and I don't remember the last time I had a cold or flu. In fact I don't remember feeling this alive. I have so much more energy now it's no longer a chore to get out of bed. I get to enjoy horseback riding with my daughter and go hiking with friends once or twice a week. I go swimming in the public pool, sit in the jacuzzi, and steam bath once a week. And I no longer feel self-conscious about my weight.

To-date I have lost over 100 pounds, my waist has shrunk from a size 46 down to a comfortable 32. Today I just eat real whole foods prepared at home. We now only go out to restaurants for special occasions. I try to buy organic foods when possible but in this economy I can't always afford it. I like to go to farmers markets and try to get local foods as much as possible.

Last year I started growing my own vegetables and now I raise chickens for healthy eggs, instead of the garbage you can find at the grocery store. Next year I plan to expand the vegetable garden and produce more of what I consume. I don't believe it's totally necessary to go to the extremes that I have in order to regain your health and lose weight. I think it boils down to changing a few habits, a willingness to learn something new, educate yourself, adapt, and just eat real whole foods. Start by picking up a few books, like the book I mentioned earlier, *The Protein Power Lifeplan*, by Mary Dan Eades, MD. and Michael R, Eades, MD.; *Why We Get Fat*, by Gary Taubes; and *The Art and Science of Low Carbohydrate Living* by Jeff Volek, PhD and Stephen Phinney, PhD. I could list more books, but these are the ones that really made an impact on my life and helped me the most.

You can find me in Tom Naughton's Facebook group, FATHEAD, helping out wherever I can. I've shared my story in the hopes that it will inspire others who struggled with their weight and health to finally reach their goal.

ELLEN KAPLAN GOFFIN

SCHAUMBURG, ILLINOIS

"I can't imagine not eating ANY grains." That's what I wrote online to Tricia, a friend who lives across the country in 2011. She had "gone paleo" and was extolling its virtues. I found it too hard to observe Passover and not eat any leavened food for a week in the spring, and considered a day or two of deprivation to be adequate. I thought it was extreme to give up a whole food group. I chose to ignore the fact that for 16 years, from 1986 to 2002, I had been a vegetarian (and for two of those years a vegan) and had indeed seen no problem with giving up whole food groups. I also thought that I was healthy and had no driving reason to try paleo as many with chronic diseases or issues do. Tricia kept sharing her successes: weight lost, muscles built, energy high. She sent links to articles, blogs, podcasts, and books. I love to learn about new things, even when I don't agree, and I pride myself on being open-minded – so I dabbled. I read a little, listened a little, sent her arguments against paleo, and even tried not eating grains for a day here and week there. She patiently explained paleo to me, and never attacked.

Then another friend, Mimi, more local, also started talking about paleo. She had joined a CrossFit gym and when she wasn't talking about that, she was talking about food. Her crossfit "box" was doing a paleo challenge. She went for it. She shared her positive results, including improved digestion.

I have two boys, ages 11 and 14. During the fall of 2011 my 11-year-old was feeling unwell. He was often tired, complaining of stomach pain, was depressed, losing his appetite, and had diarrhea. Our family doctor recommended blood tests. The test revealed that he was anemic. The doctor referred us to a pediatric gastro-intestinal group. The GI doctor told us to schedule various tests for him. During this time he was getting worse, losing significant weight, nauseated, and vomiting. We made it to the last procedure, an upper and lower endoscopy. Afterwards my husband and I were told our youngest son had Crohn's Disease.

He was admitted directly to the hospital for several nights to get him stabilized, hydrated, on steroids, and to determine a plan of action with medications. Crohn's Disease is an auto-immune disease that affects the digestive system. In my son's case, his large intestine (colon) and esophagus were affected. There is no known cure, only treatment and medication, with hope of long periods of remission. I started to research Crohn's Disease and Inflammatory Bowel Disease (IBD) in general (which includes both Crohn's Disease and Ulcerative Colitis). I found more than one first-hand account of a paleo diet putting Crohn's Disease in remission.

So now "paleo" was coming at me from multiple directions, with multiple motivations. Something Tricia had shared with me struck a chord. She told me that cattle are fed grains in order to fatten them up quickly. I actually knew that already, but in that moment the light bulb went off and I made the connection: Grains make us fat too! Of course! In February 2012 I took a plunge into the 21-Day Sugar Detox (courtesy of Diane Sanfilipo of Balanced Bites) that Tricia had done.

I have always had a sweet tooth so giving up sugar and all sweeteners was a BIG move. Sugar, in its many forms, is in so many processed foods! I learned how to avoid these items or make homemade versions. I started at "level 1" which is not strictly paleo because ½ cup of beans or rice is allowed per day. The first three days found me in a battle of wills against the sugar craving monster inside me. I wanted ice cream! Cookies! I was used to eating something "junky" and sweet almost every day, sometimes in great excess.

I persevered, and on day four it all became easy. I discovered that I only ate my ½ cup of rice about 6 days out of the 21. I was very surprised that I didn't miss bread and pasta (staples in my diet before) at all! I also discovered that my energy levels were stable throughout the day, my hunger was manageable, and my mood was consistently high. I no longer experienced low blood sugar episodes where I felt shaky and light-headed and needed food NOW. My digestion also improved. I hadn't realized it needed improvement, but once on this plan noticed I was experiencing less gas. After the detox was over I started eating a primal diet (basically a paleo diet with the inclusion of some dairy such as full fat milk, full fat Greek yogurt and grass-fed butter). I felt great! I couldn't believe it! My energy levels, both mental and physical, increased and "down" periods became shorter. As time went on, I noticed my PMS symptoms lessening dramatically. Instead of a week of cramps before and during my period, I had 1-2 days of cramps before and 1-2 days during. For the first time in years I didn't need to take over the counter pain killers! Instead of major chocolate and sugar cravings, I experienced some mild cravings. And the irritability, anxiety, and mood swings all but disappeared! I wouldn't have believed it if it didn't actually happen to me.

My exercise patterns began to change as well. I love running and was doing a lot of it (3 marathons to date) but realized my chronic cardio was not doing my body any favors. I'm one of those who did NOT lose weight training for a marathon and, in fact, sometimes gained a little. In late May I started doing CrossFit at the same box Mimi belongs to. CrossFit is so very challenging and so very fun! It is also a great place to meet like-minded people who are eating paleo or learning about it. I now do a CrossFit WOD (workout of the day) 3 times a week and walk, bike, run, or hike another 2 times a week, give or take. I feel so exuberant and youthful, and I am 44 years old!

I am still the only paleo person in my family; my husband and two boys are not on board. But I have moved them more in that direction because I am the one that prepares 95% of the food. I hope that with time, they will also see the benefits of a paleo lifestyle. My youngest is

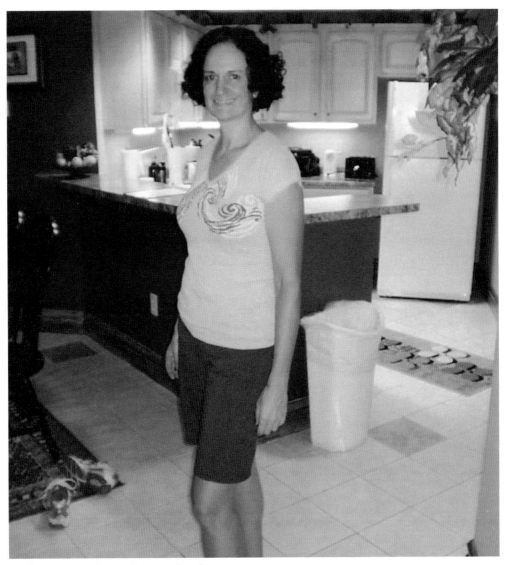

trying new foods slowly and doing his best.

I have saved the best for last. The very best "side effect" of going paleo though is the sense of freedom. I now love food without reservation! I used to have a love-hate relationship with food. I loved eating it, but I hated thinking about it. I have never had a diagnosed eating disorder but I think, like the majority of Western woman in this time in history, that I suffered from non-clinical "disordered eating." I know now that my thinking was disordered. "What should I eat?" "What do I want to eat?" "Should I eat that?" "How much fat is in that?" "How many calories are in this?" "Oh, why did I eat that?" "I should eat this but I really want that." "That will make me fat." And on and on. My thoughts about food had been torturous. I used to put myself down if I ate too much or ate the "wrong" food. I battled with myself daily, several times a day usually, about what and how much to eat. I used to weigh myself every day (okay, multiple times a day).

Guess what? Those days are now over! I love food. Food is what keeps me alive and gives me energy. Food nourishes me and enables me to do what I want to do. I eat when I am hungry.

I stop when I am full. I eat nutrient-dense foods that fill me up and make me feel good. I satisfy my hunger with protein and healthy fats and carbs, too. Certain things are off limits: no processed foods, no grains, no legumes, and little dairy. These "restrictions" (which really don't feel restrictive) do not mean I will never eat something non-paleo again. There are times I do for a special occasion, but they really are just special times that I consciously decide on and not part of my daily, or even weekly, life.

There is no price tag that can be put on this freedom!

BROOK DUBOSE

LAFAYETTE, LOUISIANA

brookd87@gmail.com

I am 25 years old, 5', 7", and weigh 155 pounds.

Before paleo my health wasn't too bad as far as I knew - although I did have a brush with suspected heart and/or brain issues when I had a tachycardic episode (my heart rate was way too high) followed by loss of consciousness ("syncopal episode") twice within three years. I had blood work done, MRIs performed, an echocardiograph, and a halter monitor for 48 hours. The results were listed as "likely vasovagal syncope." They were unable to confirm the diagnosis as they must catch an event actually happening on an EKG in order to be certain, and as much as I tried I could not force it to happen.

Fast forward 2-3 years later, I'm topping the scale at a horrifying (to me) 190 pounds. I'm fat and out of shape. All of my friends are joining local crossfit gyms and one is even training for the special forces. I was THAT guy, the token fat out of shape guy in the group. Through crossfit, my special forces friend was introduced to the paleo diet. To me this seemed absurd - he ate nothing but meat and veggies, was a stickler for salt being ADDED to his meals, and rarely if ever drank (in south Louisiana!), and the more I heard by word of mouth about it, the more I wanted to make fun of it. I even went so far as to comment: "Oh I'll just go ahead and eat like a caveman instead and eat raw meat."

Being the inquisitive person I am, with my interest and education focused in biology, I finally figured I would take a look at it. I mean my special ops friend a few short months before had weighed a staggering 230 pounds and woke up one morning and said "Uh, I think I'm going to get in shape." Next thing I know, he was down to about 170, with broad shoulders, and a six pack. So clearly whatever he was doing was working.

So I wandered into a local book store to find some books about the topic, and came across Mark Sisson's *Primal BluePrint*, Loren Cordain's *The Paleo Diet*, and Robb Wolf's *The Paleo Solution, The Original Human Diet*. I decided to go with Robb's book. The notion that this book placed on it being the "original" way of eating stuck out to me because of my interest in human evolution. Once I started reading it, I was immediately hooked. I brought it with me everywhere days until I finished it.

Then on February 15, 2011, I decided it was time to get started. Nothing complicated I reasoned – cook a large portion of meat and some veggies and away I would go. On February 16, 2011, I had a cardiologist follow up appointment after my latest syncopal episode. They ran blood work, and it was no surprise they didn't like what they saw. I informed them I had made a dietary change and I wanted to see it through. My special ops friend is the cardiologist's son - so he was aware of what I was doing. He acknowledged that it was a good method for short term weight loss, but expressed concern with the long-term health ramifications. I decided to give it a go anyway and see where it took me.

I started out at 190 pounds. March 23, 2011, I was down to 180. On April 3, 2011, I decided I would join my friends and sign up with a crossfit gym. My gym decided to form a softball team, and with all this new energy and activity level I attained, I figured why not. After I got injured and was out for three months, then life got in the way and I fell off the nutrition wagon - I was remodeling a house, and had just graduated college with a degree in biology, and started working full time. It started with rotisserie chickens and carrots, and at the worst it was fast food full of crap that made me unable to move for at least an hour.

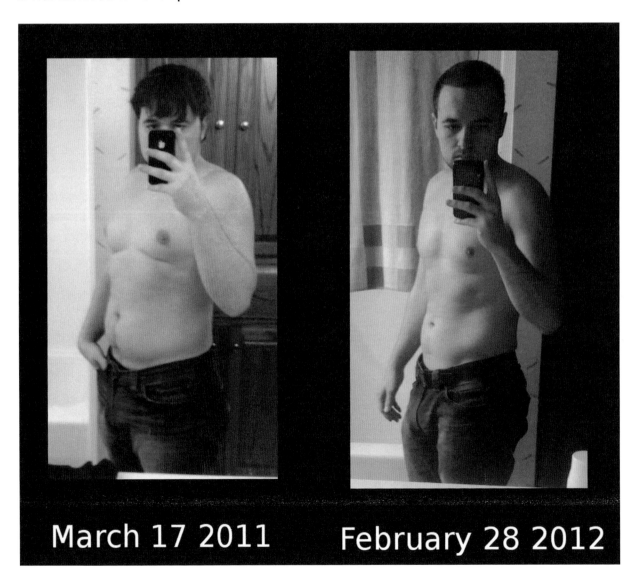

March 17 2011   February 28 2012

During that whole time, although I only gained seven pounds, my body composition took a hit, and my energy levels dropped. Nothing worth doing comes easy. It was hard to resist other people tempting me and teasing me about my radical obsession with nutrition in general.

Now I am back at it even stronger than before. I know what I am capable of. I am four weeks back into my paleo lifestyle, strict, feeling great, and back in the gym. My composition is already starting to shift back and I have lost more fat as a result. By the time this is published I will have surpassed my previous best "after" picture from March of this year.

My favorite part about this lifestyle is the community involvement, and the attention given to sustainability and food quality. The paleo community is always vigilant and always willing to question itself. When new information comes along, the paleo community is willing to reconsider their positions and, when warranted, make a change and forward that information to others in the hopes of achieving optimal health.

MEGHAN

NORTH POLE, ALASKA

My journey to better health began in July 2009. I had recently lost my son in an unexplained stillbirth and my career was on the line. My job requires a yearly fitness test, and I was not meeting the standards. I was over-weight and almost out of time. My waist was measuring at over forty four inches, which is quite large for my height of 5', 5". I had been on a specific fitness improvement program for over three years, with monthly visits to an exercise physiologist to monitor my activity level and a dietitian to help me "eat healthy."

I followed their recommendations to the letter, increasing calories, decreasing calories, more activity, less activity, weights before cardio, cardio before weights, high intensity intervals, low impact steady state, intense cardio - you name it I did it. Despite all of this, month after month I was lucky to lose one pound.

I had come to terms with the fact that I was "meant" to be fat, and that I could be healthy and fat. I embraced the "Obesity Paradox" and consoled myself with my physical abilities. My cholesterol was slightly elevated, and my blood pressure was awesome. What did it matter that going a few hours without food left me irritable and shaky? I was healthy, even though I was fat. Okay, let's be honest, at nearly 200 pounds, I was obese.

One July day, my father told me about a better way to eat based on our time-proven genetic code and years of adaptation. "Eat like a caveman," he told me. "The dietitian will ream me!" I replied. Really? No grains? No beans? No potatoes? This man was clearly out of his mind.

It was about a month before I saw him again – and in that time he lost seven inches from his waist and twenty seven pounds! I was astonished. That day I became paleo, eating the foods our ancestors ate to the best of my ability. I ate most of my food in the form of meats, vegetables and fruits. I kept almonds on hand at work, along with homemade beef jerky and

REAL bacon. I ate lots of fresh vegetables and fruits from local farm stands. It was amazing how great it felt to finally eat healthy. Not the standard way of eating based on the Food Pyramid or according to what a dietitian thought was best. These were honest to goodness nourishing foods.

Over time I found myself reaching more for stricter paleo choices. Some people say I was eating low carbohydrate and that is why I lost weight - but it definitely wasn't low carb according to diets geared at that goal. I ate/eat over 100 grams of carbohydrate a day, losing weight best at 125 or so.

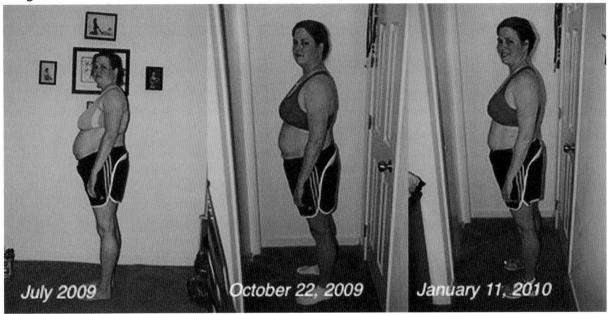

July 2009   October 22, 2009   January 11, 2010

And my weight loss was great! Ten pounds in the first month and by three months I had lost just over thirty pounds! I was excited about that, but even better was the 12+ inches of stubborn belly fat! In all the time I was trying to get fit while eating grains, I only lost about 2 inches total! With paleo I lost over 10 inches from my abdomen in just about three months.

I was even told at my next fitness exam that the person in charge of the program would probably request I be measured again because she wouldn't believe I could lose that many inches so quickly. After the first two weeks of my new lifestyle I also lost the horrible pain in my feet cause by plantar fasciitis, knee and ankle joint pain. It took a year for me to notice that I no longer required breakfast and I could go hours without food and never feel angry, irritable or lightheaded. It was such a relief from being a slave to food. Adopting this healthy lifestyle helped me go from 190+ pounds to 150 pounds, from a size 22 pants to a size 10-12. It helped me pass my fitness test, improved my overall cholesterol, saved me from years of chronic pain AND saved my career.

CHARALAMPOS ZOIS TILAS

REGENSBURG, GERMANY

babis@me.com

My name is Charalampos Zois Tilas. My friends call me Babis. I was 32 years old when I started with my new lifestyle. I started paleo almost two years ago, in October 2010. Before paleo I weighed about 226 pounds at a height of 5', 8.5". I didn't have serious health problems, but I didn't feel really that my body was really healthy.

Every time I tried to participate in a sport, like cycling or running, to lose weight, it lasted only a couple of minutes until I was exhausted. Most of the time, I ordered pizza or similar junk food right afterwards.

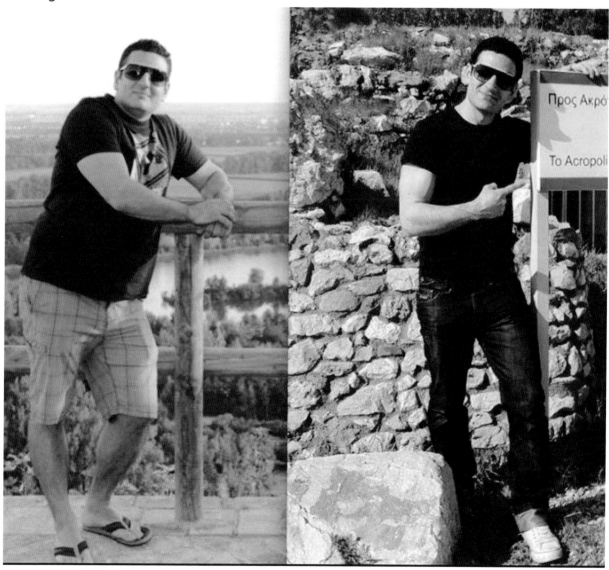

My total cholesterol was over 300 and the ratios were even worse. My doctor kept telling me that I needed to lose weight, but I had no idea how to do that. This kept on going until I asked a friend of mine, Markus Prygoda, to help me. He was always in a great shape and knew a lot about nutrition.

He told me about the paleo lifestyle, and said I should give it a try. He explained all the basics and wrote me a meal plan for the first couple of weeks. Before that, I was eating a lot of bread, tons of sweets, chips, ice cream, and I drank coke.

Well, October 10th 2010 was the first day in my new life. From that day on, I ate and still eat a lot of meat, vegetables, and have ditched all the processed foods. I drink coffee with a little coconut milk and I also drink a lot of water. No juices, not even fresh ones, because of the excessive fructose content.

It was not easy as it might sound. The first days were terrible. I craved bread so badly. I would do anything for bread. And that was the most difficult part of that change. I felt like an addict the first days. Two to three weeks later, I noticed that my pants were getting looser - or was it me getting thinner?! That encouraged me a lot.

After one month I had lost almost 18 pounds, and I wanted more! My family and friends were concerned because of the high amount of meat and fat I was eating.

Now, almost two years later, I weigh 169.4 pounds, and my total cholesterol is at 190 and the ratios are fantastic. I bike a lot now, can run a 10k without any problems and I do crossfit.

Thanks go to Markus Prygoda for helping me and for all the support, even when he was out the country. Thank you!

SIMONE SHIFNADEL

SAN FRANCISCO, CALIFORNIA

zenbellysf@gmail.com , zenbellyblog.com , zenbellycatering.com

My paleo transformation might be less dramatic than some, but the change I've felt has been quite profound.

Although I haven't had any serious chronic health problems, my health has been less than optimal for my entire life: colds twice a year, lethargy, acne, headaches, brain fog, blood sugar crashes, general malaise, mild depression, and pretty intense mood swings.

I did not seek medical attention for any of these issues. I do not seek out western medicine unless I have a physical injury.

These conditions were at their absolute worst when I was between the ages of 20-26, the years that I was a vegetarian/pescetarian. I was in a relationship with someone who couldn't eat dairy, so I was also eating a LOT of soy products that we had in the house as dairy substitutes. I was also working in a vegetarian restaurant, and while there, ate things like seitan. The seitan rueben was my favorite lunch: wheat gluten on wheat bread. Yes, I was the angry chef who sometimes threw pans. I was a pretty unhappy person in general. I was about 155 pounds at 5'7". Not fat by any means, but heavy for me.

I started eating meat right around the time I got out of that relationship. I lost about ten pounds without really trying (certainly not by exercising) and noticed a definite improvement in my mood. I was far from paleo at this point, and for the next 5 years as well. I ate whatever I wanted, but as a chef I have never been much of a packaged foods junkie. I was, however, consuming massive amounts of gluten. And the headaches, lethargy, frequent colds, skin breakouts, and brain fog remained. It was getting to the point that I was fairly certain that something was wrong with me.

The next few years strongly resembled a roller coaster, and involved massage school, new job, new relationships, moving from upstate New York to Massachusetts for a mere 6 months, and more than my fair share of emotional turmoil. The only "sensible" solution was to give away my stuff and drive to California with my dog, clothes, and chef knives.

In 2007, shortly after moving to California, I began to see a chiropractor who did food sensitivity testing as part of a holistic approach to health. I had a feeling that gluten was an issue for a while, but being a chef, the idea of having to eliminate something from my diet was almost too awful to comprehend. Naturally, gluten showed up on the test results. So I eliminated it. Well, sort of. I made an effort to cut it out of my everyday life, but still had a slice of pizza when I was in New York, or sometimes a sandwich. I still used the soy sauce in sushi places. Even without being diligent about getting the gluten out, I felt a hundred times better.

I still got frequent breakouts, colds at least twice a year, and was hungry often. If I didn't eat before my blood sugar crashed, I basically fell apart.

It was only about two years ago that I first heard about paleo. I was enrolled in an online nutrition program that covered several different diets, and paleo was one of them. We covered the pros and cons as we did every other diet we studied. I didn't come away from it feeling that paleo was the answer.....after all, whole grains are healthy, and saturated fat is bad, right?!?

Then I read Robb Wolf's *The Paleo Solution*, and watched Dr. Terry Wahls' account of reversing her Multiple Sclerosis with a nutrient-dense diet. And I started to read labels more and more - it started to become clear that there weren't many things with a label that I wanted to be eating.

I've been mostly paleo for about a year and a half, and seem to be getting closer to completely paleo as time goes on. I'm about 95% paleo at home. It's how I cook. When I'm away from home, I lighten up a bit. I'm not religious about this way of life - gluten is a definite no, no matter what. There is no cheating on that, and I get very upset if I accidentally get

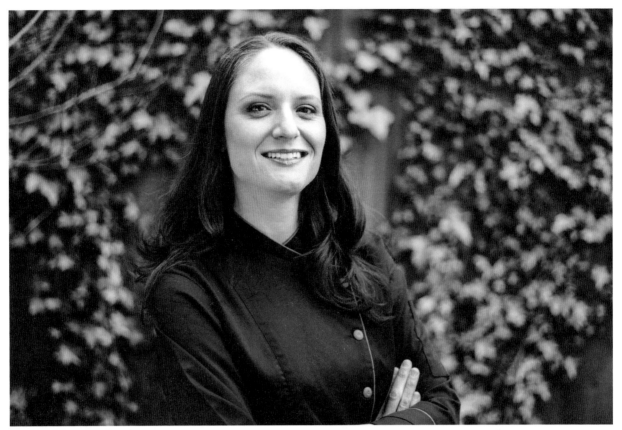

glutened. If I go out for sushi, I will eat some white rice in my favorite rolls. If I go to someone's house for dinner and they worked very hard to make me a gluten-free meal that's not exactly paleo, I will be polite about it and grateful that someone cooked for me. I also happen to be friends with some extremely talented gluten-free bakers, and if they give me a loaf of gluten-free sourdough, I'll enjoy it with some cioppino. I was in dairy denial until about two months ago, and continued to consume cream in my coffee, full fat yogurt, and ice cream. I have recently made the dairy-skin connection, and am positive that the frequent breakouts are dairy related, so bye-bye dairy. That has been the hardest thing to cut out. I don't miss grains, I definitely don't miss beans, and I can easily curb the sweets. But dairy! I do miss dairy.

So what's left of my long list of less than ideal health conditions?

No more brain fog. No more lethargy. I can't remember the last time I got a cold. My blood sugar is stable, and when I go hours without eating, no one around me fears for their life. As long as I don't eat dairy, I don't break out. I get a headache once in a while, but it's usually the result of neck tension rather than toxic food choices. I'm still an emotional person, but I'm 100% sure that no diet will ever change that. The last item for me to tackle in this paleo life is to conquer my hatred for exercise. I know the importance of it, but can't seem to find an activity that I enjoy. I am, however, a good example for those who shun the high fat diet, and are sure that eating fat will make them fat. I just point to myself and say "Avocado! Coconut! Bacon! Size 6, and I don't exercise!"

Another great benefit of this new lifestyle is the way it has impacted my career. My catering company has evolved along with me, and is now a 100% gluten-free operation, specializing in paleo cuisine. I am in the process of opening up a gluten-free shared kitchen in San Francisco, with paleo meals to go. This way of life has fueled the fire, and made me a more ambitious person. My job is to provide people with food that I feel great about feeding them. In the process, I get to support local family farms and ranches. How great is that? Check out my websites: zenbellyblog.com and zenbellycatering.com !

KARL ZAPF

MECHANICSVILLE, VIRGINIA

I have always considered myself to be a healthy person. Throughout school, I participated in team sports like football, hockey, and track. Later, I became an avid mountain biker and finished the "Chequamagon 40" three times – a 40-mile mountain bike race held each year in the Hayward, Wisconsin area. However, in 2009 I found myself heading for trouble. At age 52, my weight was approaching 300 pounds. There were long periods of time when I would not step on the scale, so I don't really know how high my weight went. I was also suffering debilitating back pain, along with many other small ailments that I attributed to my age.

Because I am 6′, 5″ tall, I carried my excess weight well and people didn't really see me as obese. Unfortunately I began to suffer excruciating back pain on a daily basis. I saw a chiropractor who took x-rays and told me he found it hard to believe I could walk at all. I had degenerating discs in my neck and herniated discs in my lower back. I missed more work during 2009 and early 2010 than ever before because of my back condition. I lived on a steady stream of pain relievers…Advil, Aleve, and eventually prescription muscle relaxers. Once home from work in the evening, I would drink a few beers to ease the pain and lay on the couch with my feet up until I fell asleep. Eventually, my wife would shoo me off to bed where I found I could not get comfortable.

At the end of 2009, in desperation, I saw an orthopedic surgeon. I am so thankful he did not recommend surgery, because I would have done anything to try to feel better. Instead, he prescribed physical therapy, which I began in 2010. I asked my physical therapist if it would help me of I lost weight, but she said "no, you aren't that heavy." Looking around at the other patients in the physical therapist's office, I felt pretty good. My weight seemed normal compared to many of the others. While the physical therapy helped a little, the main benefit was that it kept me from doing anything drastic about my back pain (like getting surgery). I didn't know it, but real help was right around the corner.

During this time, I stopped riding my mountain bike and took up hiking as a more "appropriate" activity for someone my weight. This was on the advice of my chiropractor, and I knew he was right. Due to my back issues, each downward push of the bike pedal resulted in a searing pain. I felt I had no strength to push the pedals. So I was done with bike riding, at least for the time being. Unfortunately, throughout 2009 and 2010, even hiking became difficult. Any step could trigger nerve pain running up and down my leg. I even fell down on the trail during one hike because I just lost all strength in my leg. I felt like my broken and battered 50+ year old body could not handle the types of play activities I still wanted to do.

As we moved into 2011, my wife and I decided to try eating a lower carbohydrate diet. We both read *Good Calories, Bad Calories,* by Gary Taubes. I had succeeded in losing weight before eating low-carb, so we started to try it again. But I was still eating a lot of bread. Typically I would skip breakfast and have a low-calorie frozen meal, plus chips, fruit, and a sweet treat for lunch. At home in the afternoon, I would snack on cheese and crackers, or chips, until dinner. I typically ended each day with a slice of bread and peanut butter. The small changes we made to be "low-carb" were not having much effect. We were eating a lot of low-carb garbage instead of eating real food, and hunger could easily de-rail my plan to cut out my evening bread and peanut butter snack.

Our change to paleo was gradual, and I don't remember exactly when in 2011 I began to think of my diet as "paleo". On the recommendation of friends, I began reading Mark Sisson's website, Mark's Daily Apple, and taking away ideas to try. In late spring, my wife and I decided to give up grains and see what would happen. We also stopped buying salad dressing at the store (avoiding soybean oil), and stopped eating legumes. By summer of 2011, we went paleo and I started to see the weight come off. In fact, over the twelve month period from May 2011 to May 2012, I lost 55 pounds. I even exercised, and I still enjoyed a beer or two on the weekends.

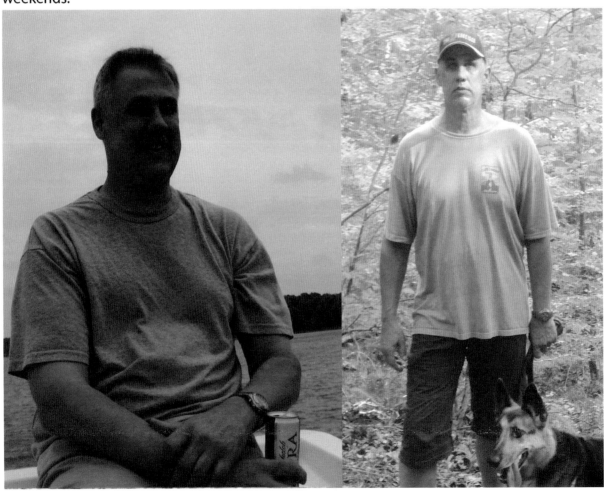

I did not enter into a paleo lifestyle thinking I would resolve my health problems. I wasn't even sure I would lose weight. Not only did my new diet improve my back pain, but it also helped now I recognize that grains, processed foods, and sugar were the causes of a long-term health issues including Irritable Bowel Syndrome (IBS). I had never seen a doctor for it (real men stay away from the doctors, right?), but I had suffered bouts of gas and diarrhea every few days for my entire adult life. Now I can go weeks without any flare-up. I can also hike long and difficult mountain trails completely pain-free without falling down, and haven't missed work due to my back issues in over a year. This spring, I went on a bike ride for the first time since 2009. Pain medications are a thing of the past.

I love to cook, and eating paleo allows me to try new recipes every week. On a typical day, I will have a breakfast frittata with egg, sausage, peppers and onions. Lunch is leftovers from dinner the night before, along with fruit and a handful of nuts. Dinner is grass-fed beef, wild-caught salmon, or pastured chicken along with a salad and possibly a sweet potato. My wife makes all of our salad dressings and mayonnaise from scratch using good quality olive oil. On the weekends, I really cook. We have tried a paleo-version of Crawfish Fettuccine, Oysters Rockefeller, Tacos de Lengua, and many other great recipes. We like to pair our creations with craft beers (technically not Paleo, but very tasty) and good wines. Amazingly, I find I can eat whatever I want so long as I avoid grains and legumes. My weight stays constant, my back and bowels feel good, and I feel young again – at almost 55! I am no longer concerned that my body won't support the play activities I want to do. I am a new man.

MONIQUE

ALGOMA MILLS, ONTARIO, CANADA

I am 43 years old. Before I went paleo, I was overweight, over 165 pounds, and out of shape and tired...all the time. In high school and college, I had played a lot of volleyball and badminton. In the summer months, I played baseball. I loved being active. I had to give it all up back in 2000 (roughly) because of my arthritis, and I gained weight. Plus my diet was your typical SAD diet, carbs on top of carbs. Not a lot of fresh fruit and not a lot of fresh vegetables. And the meat was usually processed and battered.

Let's take a moment to go through all my medical conditions:

- I was diagnosed with colitis in 2002, but had IBS (Irritable Bowel Syndrome) for many years before that. I took medications for a short time (salofalk enemas), which helped keep the flare ups under control. In 2006, I had a major flare up which hospitalized me. I was dehydrated and had migraines. I wasn't eating because I didn't want to deal with the stomach cramps. Then I started salofalk suppositories and later was prescribed Asacol.

- I was diagnosed with arthritis in the 90s, and it grew worse over time. It was a challenge to get out of bed, walk down stairs, open a can, shift gears, and even to brush my teeth. I could not function. The pain was more than I could handle. I was prescribed Vioxx and took that for at least 5 years. In 2002 I was given a prescription for Methotrexate and told it would help my future' arthritis conditions.

- I also had psoriasis, since I was a child. There were patches all over me, mostly on my scalp. I was prescribed Betnovate cream to treat it.

- My migraines started in college. They seemed to follow my hormonal patterns and only popped up around my cycle. In 2005, I started taking Imitrex to treat them. When they happened, 1-2 times a month, they were so bad that I had to miss a day and a half of work.

In January of 2011 a friend of mine Troy V. had been sending informational messages to me on Facebook about paleo. I ignored most of them. Eventually, I got chatting with him because my symptoms were not getting better, and I was looking for answers. He simplified paleo for me and it all made perfect sense - the connection between food and inflammation. It finally clicked. I wanted to know more, and joined some groups on Facebook, including the International Paleo Movement Group (http://is.gd/paleogroup), and this enabled me to talk to may others about their successes.

Without Troy I never would have began this journey...and I would still be suffering. In March of 2011, I decided to make a conscious effort to apply paleo to my life.

I'll admit, it wasn't an easy transition. We grew up with fast, convenient food. Having to change that mindset has - and still is - taking time. Learning to shop and think ahead has proved to be a challenge. Grocery shopping, packing lunches, late suppers on busy weeknights...every day provides a new challenge, but every day I'm learning. But now I can say that I have beaten the grain demons! I don't fight any urges anymore because they don't exist! I can go by the chip and soda pop isle at the grocery store and not desire any of it as I proudly look down at my cart full of fresh fruit, vegetables, and meat!!!

Today I weigh 115 pounds.

My colitis is ongoing, but I do not deal with cramping or 'needing to go.' It is much less severe and more manageable – and I am taking half the dosage of medication that I took five year ago. My Arthritis is sooooo much better! I've started to play sports again...and work out!! Losing weight helped tremendously (35 pounds lost in the first 6 months of paleo!). I wasn't in so much pain. I feel fit and active. In your face arthritis!! I have cut my Methotrexate by over half and plan to continue reducing my intake. I started to notice a change with my arthritis almost immediately. My migraines are far less active. I still keep the Imitrex on hand just in case. When and if they happen, they no longer last for days. My colitis isn't quite as severe, but I still deal with it daily. It's really hit or miss. Food sometimes affects it. I can never find a pattern. I just know that with paleo I feel somewhat in control.

My overall health feels different than it did 2 years ago. I can't explain it. I'm not tired all the time. And I feel good about my body.

My family and friends didn't (and still don't) quite understand. I explain to those who ask. But they see the results - physically, the weight loss, and mentally, I'm just a happier person! My overall mood and outlook on life has changed, and people notice that. Paleo has helped me change my attitude toward foods and I feel like I have been armed with great powers. I've

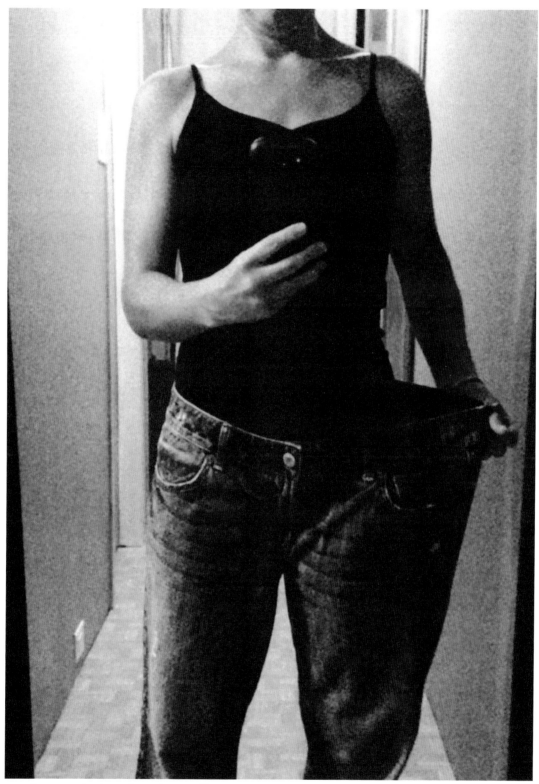

come to the conclusion that they will never truly understand unless they take that step and experience paleo for themselves.

When someone asks, I take the time and tell them about paleo...I tell them that paleo has

GIVEN ME MY LIFE BACK!!! I can't express how much better I feel because of how, and what I eat.

Paleo is not a restricted diet in the common sense of the words. Once you start to feel and see results, you know it's worth it. All that extra time prepping food, or extra money you pay for fresh food – the benefits are immeasurable. There is no amount of medication that can make you feel that way.

ZACK

OCEAN, NEW JERSEY

The Christmas before I turned 25, I got a gym membership. As a poor 20 something, I was determined to get the biggest bang for my buck from it. I talked to a friend who is a nutritionist about maximizing my weight loss and strength building. I am 5', 10.5" and at the time, weighed 205 pounds. He told me to cut down on carbs and alcohol. So I did. I moderately cut back on my carb intake and lost a fair amount of weight in the first month.

But I started to plateau, so I went back to him and told him. That's when he laid the paleo diet on me. After being primed with cutting back on my carb intake, the paleo diet made absolute sense to me and I was excited to try it. Over the next 5 months, I dropped to 190 pounds based solely on a simplified understanding of the diet. This was in 2007, so the online resources didn't exist like they do now and there certainly wasn't a large community like there is now. After a 6 month stint on the paleo diet, I got married. My new wife wasn't paleo. This made it hard to stick to the diet and I was off and on for the next few years.

In late November of 2009, we had our son and for the next year my wife didn't lose any of the weight she had put on during pregnancy. She had had enough of being heavy and was determined to make a change. So I helped her get onto a strict paleo diet (even though I didn't join her). She lost 50 pounds in the first 3 months *before* joining a gym. Since then, she has toned and shaped her way to a better weight/body than she had for years before. After a year of watching her success, I was inspired to get back in gear.

It was December 2011 and I realized in six months, we would go to the beach and I would have to explain how it was possible a woman that looked like she did could possibly be with someone who looked like I did. But I decided to put it off through the holiday season.

It was now the beginning of 2012 and my 30th birthday was fast approaching in February. I started doing some more research online for more paleo information and to my amazement the web had exploded with resources that hadn't been there when I first found paleo. Not only that, but there were Facebook groups and Google+ discussions! I quickly began communicating with people as much as I could and built a plan to get myself back on the paleo lifestyle, but this time for good.

By March 1, 2012 I was ready to implement it. In the first 3 months I dropped from 210 pounds to 178 pounds. My waist shrank from 38" to 33". I am now at 185, and my waist is 32", and it's only 7 months since I started back up.

My mild psoriasis isn't gone, but it is far better. I don't get seasonal allergies anymore either, nor have I gotten a common cold since I started. I have more energy than I know what to do with most days. Results from my most recent doctor visit in May were positive, including my cholesterol analysis.

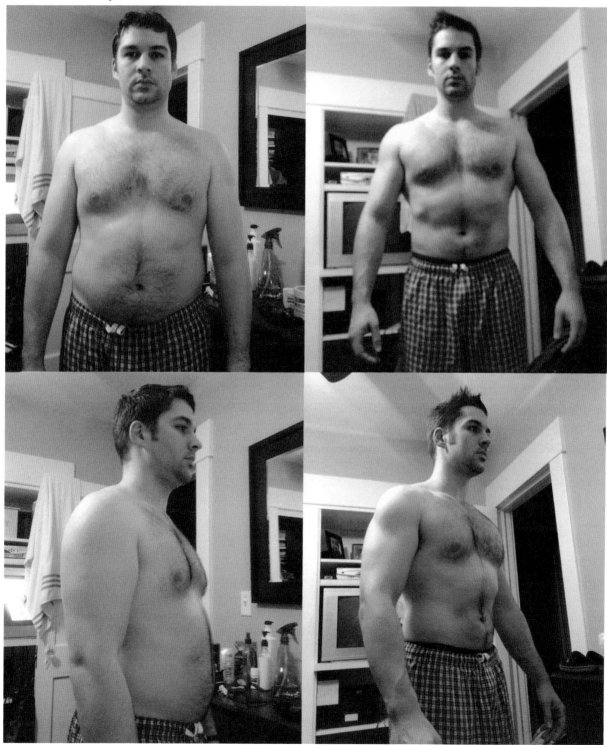

Before I went paleo the first time, I was a pretty normal eater. I ate home cooked meals, but also would from time to time have sub sandwiches, ice cream, pie, cookies, soda, etc. I wasn't just eating garbage, but I certainly wasn't avoiding it either. Now I am eating meat, veggies, fruit (mainly after workouts), nuts as a snack or as a flour substitution, and starchy tubers (mainly after workouts).

I allow myself a handful of "cheat" days for special or traditional occasions, but I don't generally *want* to eat that kind of food. I have shifted my paradigm to believe that it's literally poison – which makes it hard to want to consume. That might sound extreme, but it helps keep me focused on eating the right stuff during the rare bad craving.

There are challenges to this lifestyle, especially in the beginning. First is the low carb flu which for me lasted about 2.5 weeks. From my experience the first time, it's important to note that living with a non-paleo eater is quite difficult in terms of adherence. Being aware of it ahead of time is the best way to combat it. Either you will have to cook for yourself or find things to make that are "secretly" paleo where whomever you are feeding doesn't even realize it.

Also know that you will be tempted at first. There is no way around it. Trucks drive ice cream around your neighborhood, relatives make cakes and cookies and pies, they sell sausage sandwiches at sporting events. If you want to give in to temptation from time to time, I think it is fine. My goal is not to go overboard and limit the cheat to that one day.

My wife is much closer to 80/20 than I am. Everyone will find their own balance. If I were doing it all over again for the first time, this is the advice I would give myself: (1) take a before picture because you will not believe the difference a few months makes, (2) be very strict for the first 30 days, and (3) find like minded people to talk about it with as a sort of support group, even if though the internet.

The biggest downside to the lifestyle is all the new clothes you may have to buy. I remain convinced that the guidelines of the paleo lifestyle are good for everyone. It's framework is specific enough to tell you what to avoid, but broad enough to accommodate different eating styles.

JENN TYLER

WILTON, IOWA

onemomagainstthegrain.blogspot.com

Before paleo, my diet consisted mostly of pasta with creamy sauces made with low fat ingredients, boneless/skinless chicken breasts, lots of sugar treats, fast food and pizza. I was a long distance runner and felt the extra calories I burned running so many miles would make up for the poor food choices. I suffered from piriformis syndrome and posterior tibial tendonitis, common running injuries, brought on by overtraining, and went to see a chiropractor who specialized in athletes. The piriformis syndrome was pinching my sciatic nerve and causing a lot of pain in my foot and hip. The chiropractor performed Active Release

Techniques (ART) on me twice a week in an attempt to reduce the inflammation in my pirforimis to release my sciatic nerve. She was also treating my posterior tibial tendonitis with ART. I also had depression and anxiety disorder, and I was seeing a psychiatrist for meds every 1-3 months and seeing a psychologist for "talk therapy" monthly.

I discovered the paleo lifestyle in early 2011 at the age of 31, while I was training for numerous half marathons. My chiropractor looked at me one day after about 5 or 6 months of ART Treatment and said "There is nothing else I can do for you. You need to change your diet to see any more relief" for the running injuries. She suggested I start following a more paleo diet. She explained what paleo was. I said that I didn't think I could do that – it felt too extreme to me. She then recommended that I at least remove gluten, sugar, and dairy from my diet for two weeks and see how I felt. She even guaranteed I'd lose 10 pounds. So, I gave it a shot. I got gluten-free this, gluten-free that. I followed her rules for 6 days, and already had lost 8 pounds, and started to feel some pain relief with my piriformis syndrome and tibial tendonitis. But I didn't stick with it, and my weight loss didn't stick around either. And my piriformis syndrome and tibial tendonitis pain returned.

I limped through all 6 of my half marathons that year, and called it a season. I went about trying to lose weight the Conscious Wellness route, and was getting nowhere. I studied many different diets and worked hard to make them work, but it didn't get me anywhere. It was quite frustrating. I had a few friends who were doing paleo, but I thought there was NO WAY I could give up my pasta – I mean, I'm a runner! Runners need pasta!

On March 5, 2012 I decided to take the full paleo plunge. I was going to go full throttle into Mark Sisson's book, *The Primal Blueprint*, and see what could happen. After reading *The Primal Blueprint*, I was intrigued. I wanted to continue reading, so I also read Dr. Davis' *Wheat Belly* and decided wheat was just all around bad and there was no going back. I was not going to eat wheat again because I was fearful of the damage it could do. I also read Melissa and Dallas Hartwig's *It Starts with Food*.

These days I am paleo and my breakfast consists of eggs and bacon! Imagine that! BACON! I used to avoid bacon because of the high calorie content. Now I relish it because of the high fat content! Being paleo, I know that I don't have to stress about calories if I don't want to. My dinner looks like a juicy ribeye steak with fresh steamed veggies or a baked sweet potato. Lunch is usually leftovers from dinner. We no longer eat anything that comes packaged in a box or that has been prepared in a factory. All of our foods are fresh meats, fresh vegetable and fresh fruits.

The hardest part about making the switch was seeing my family eat old favorites – pizza, lasagna, etc. – and I overcame this by converting my family as well. My husband, 5-year old son and 2 year old daughter now eat the same dinners I do. The kids sometimes complain and ask for their old favorites, like chicken nuggets and pizza, and sometimes we compromise and let them enjoy them, but those days are fewer and further between as they are adjusting to the new way of eating and seeing great results.

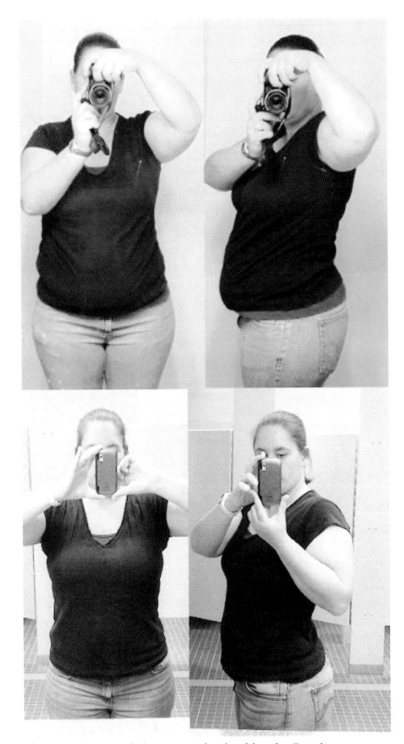

After making the change to Primal, I've never looked back. Don't get me wrong, I have slipped a couple of times and ate a cupcake at my niece's 4th birthday, have eaten a Tombstone with my family, and have gone out to eat and have eaten non-paleo things… but, I recognize my slip and get back on track. I know that eating paleo makes me feel SO much better both physically and mentally and that always brings me back.

Since March, I've lost a total of 35 pounds! I have taken 26.5 inches off of my body. I have gone from a tight size 16 to a size 12 that fits comfortably. I am now wearing jeans I haven't worn since before I got pregnant with my son 6 years ago!

Even more important than the weight loss is the fact I was finally able to stop taking antidepressants. I was taking three different medications to help control my moods. Since going paleo, I have not needed them and the doctor discontinued my prescriptions. My depression is gone as long as I stay the course and remain true to paleo eating. My piriformis syndrome still gets fired up when I run, but it no longer sidelines me because my body recovers more quickly. My posterior tibial tendonitis is completely gone. One of the more surprising things is that my exercise has been cut back dramatically! Instead of running 5 or more miles 3x per week, all I do now is walk for 45 minutes 5x per week over lunch. I am starting to gear up for another half marathon season, but I expect this time around to be MUCH different. For starters, I'm much lighter which will be less stress on my body. Running is SO much easier now. I've even ventured into barefoot running which is much more comfortable than running in shoes.

The turning point for me was when I went from being skeptical and started seeing the results that were possible with this paleo lifestyle. Once I saw results I hadn't seen with all my other failed attempts, I was sold. I am fully committed to this lifestyle! As I was reading Mark Sisson's book, I kept thinking "Yeah right! Effortless weight loss?!?", but it's absolutely true! And the change has been so easy! I love the foods I am eating! And no one is missing anything that we used to have before because we all have new favorites that we ask for regularly instead of asking for pizza or fast food!

I love my new lifestyle and I am currently reading *Primal Body Primal Mind* by Nora T. Gedgaudas and learning so much more. Reading and learning has been paramount to my transformation.

JOHANNES KWELLA

BERLIN, GERMANY

paleojay@gmail.com

I'm 27 years old. I discovered paleo 2 ½ years ago, while searching for the perfect nutritional solution was for me.

I weigh 180 pounds. I didn't think I suffered from any medical conditions, but after starting paleo, not 100% but 80/20, I felt so different! I gained a huge amount of energy, fitness, and agility throughout the day! No afternoon naps or tiredness. My bodily inflammation dramatically decreased, I am sleeping better, and I stopped having joint pain!

I first heard about paleo from Dallas and Melissa Hartwig's Whole9 website. They got me started on it and later I read Dr. Cordain's *The Paleo Diet* and Robb Wolf's *The Paleo Solution*. After reading all of this, I was sure that paleo was the right nutritional choice.

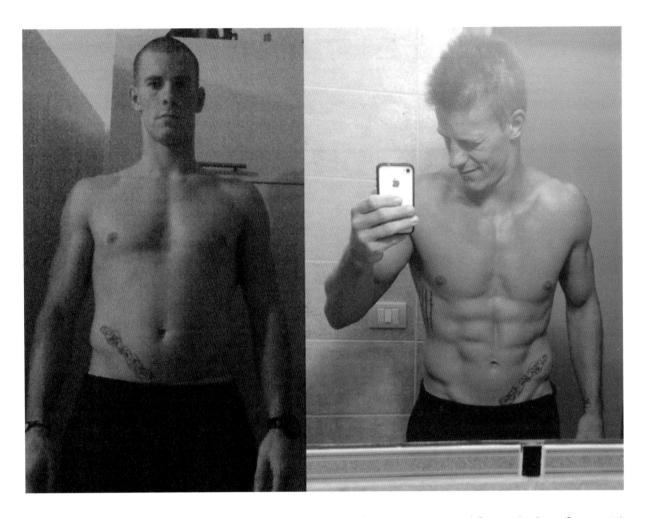

I used to typically eat all kinds of meats (usually the cheapest, minimal fat and a lot of protein) and "healthy" grains as whole wheat products which I ate every 2-3 hours. I ate everything that is considered healthy.

Now I only eat 2-3 meals in an 8 hour time frame, and fast the remaining 16 hours. On heavy training days, I have up to 2 pounds of potatoes or sweet potatoes, with high protein and moderate fat added. On other days, I will have high fat, high protein, and fewer carbs. I eat scrambled eggs, grass fed beef, pork/bacon, poultry, lots of fresh and frozen veggies, salads, and a lot of fruits. My favorite part of all of this is that I can eat a huge meal in one sitting and not feel hungry for 8 hours. There is much less preparation, and I am getting so many more nutrients than I was before.

The hardest part was the beginning! Once you are in to it, it becomes easier to keep going.

My family isn't paleo but that's OK – I am doing this for me.

A. D.

AURORA, COLORADO

I was diagnosed with Multiple Sclerosis (MS) at age 30, months after having my second child and moving cross country. My left side became so weak I dropped my baby one time (fortunately catching her midair) and dragged my left leg. My fatigue was so great that I needed a nap after showering. From February 2005 until April 2011 I took my $20,000 a year MS injectable prescription drug and still had new MS symptoms, and even 5-7 new MS lesions (unusable tissue) on my brain every year.

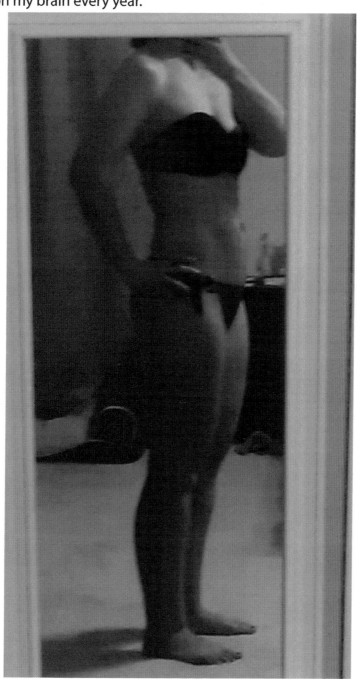

In April 2011 I ran into an old friend who convinced me to try going gluten free for 30 days to combat my MS fatigue. I resisted at first, then realized that I had nothing to lose. After 30 days passed gluten-free, it was time for my biannual appointment with my MS neurologist.

I told him about my new diet, admitting that I thought is was bullshit, and not worth maintaining. In no uncertain terms he said that I should remain gluten free and he passionately recommended that I try going paleo too. That scared me to death! I had only committed to 30 days and now the doctor wanted me to restrict more, and for longer? I hadn't even noticed a positive change from being gluten free. The next morning, I defiantly made instant oatmeal, and within ten minutes of eating the oatmeal, my lap went NUMB! I instantly realized that I could avoid the numbness from avoiding gluten!

Over several months I gradually incorporated more paleo meals into my family's diet. Over time I felt better, stronger, and less fatigued! I started volunteering at the kids' school. I accomplished more in the house and even decided to go back to work for the first time in eleven years. Six months ago I started doing crossfit twice a week. Admittedly, I feel the effects of the intense exercise for a day or two afterward but I'm getting stronger and am able to tolerate more and more in all areas of my life.

After fourteen months of (80%) Paleo, I had the best MRI since being diagnosed with MS seven years earlier. Instead of my "normal" 5-7 new lesions, my neurologist was shocked that I only had "one TINY lesion." Paleo IS a way of life and I will never want to go back to my SAD ways again.

KAREN PENDERGRASS

MARIA DEL REY, CALIFORNIA

www.thepaleofondation.org

Before 2008, I never cared much about food, food politics, farm animals, or sustainability. But then something happened to me, something so devastating that when I unraveled the answers to my near-demise I became so pissed off that I began to delve deep into those issues. What happened? I got sick.

Not "kinda sorta sick"… it was the type of sick that had doctors scratching their heads in confusion, telling me it was unlikely that I would ever have kids, and that if I didn't get better I would end up living in a hospital or dying.

And this all sounded like bullshit to me because from what I had understood, I was doing all of the right things to take care of my body: I quit smoking the year before (after a 10 year habit) and I quit drinking alcohol except for in very small amounts on special occasions. I even began a new good habit: exercise. I exercised *all of the time*. I exercised at least once a day for an entire hour, most of the time for 2 hours. On some days I spent my time with a personal trainer (who later ended up saving my life when all she was trying to do was help my mother with her allergies). It's funny - and nothing short of a miracle - how these things worked themselves out.

I ate whole wheat bread, drank skim milk, and I didn't eat red meat. I bought fish and chicken from the grocery store because I knew that I needed some protein. As a recovering Vegetarian, that was a huge step for me. I also ate soy-protein bars because they contained a minimal amount of calories, and were "cruelty-free." Well, almost cruelty-free - the taste was torturous.

I was diligent about brushing and flossing my teeth, drinking water, and from what anyone could tell I was in excellent shape and in excellent health. I was 110 pounds, size 0, 5'5", and relatively toned. And I worked hard to keep myself that way. I looked healthy on the outside. Unfortunately, looks can be deceiving.

October 31st, 2008 was the first day that I looked as unhealthy as I actually was. It was also the first Halloween in my *entire* life that I didn't celebrate. It's hard to explain what a big deal that was to me, unless you knew that this is one out of the two days a year that I plan for months in advance.

I didn't go out that night because the costume that I had planned to wear didn't fit, and neither did my shoes. Imagine what it would look like if the Stay-Pufft marshmallow from Ghostbusters was 7 months pregnant. Got the picture in your head? Ok. That was me. That's why I didn't go out.

The next morning when I got out of bed I was dizzy with a headache, and when I got up it hurt just to *walk*. For months this pain continued and worsened, along with all sorts of new symptoms. The one in particular that made no sense was that I was gaining weight--*quickly*. So naturally I began to eat like a bird and exercise more, but despite my grandest of efforts I continued to gain weight. So I saw a physician.

She sucked. This moron explained to me that the weight gain was simply because I was taking in too many calories, and not making enough caloric expenditures - you know, the whole calories in-calories out theory. When I told her my exercise routine and my newly-formed eating habits along with my weight gain, she dismissed me completely. She explained to that I was having what she called "psychosomatic manifestations" which she blamed on "emotional stress." To be honest, she was right about the stress. I was stressed from incessantly trying to tell her that her calories-in calories-out theory was complete bullshit, trying to get some sort of validation or answer for my condition.

Fast-forward about 6 months, 30 some-odd doctor visits, and 30 pounds later. I no longer had menses, I experienced daily swelling of my legs, hands, feet and face, I couldn't wear shoes except for flip-flops, I couldn't walk, I couldn't feel my legs, and my skin hurt to the touch like I had a sunburn. I slept 20-36 hours straight and was only awake while pumping my veins full of coffee and RedBull. I was a listless zombie. I was in a fog and I couldn't focus for the life of me. I had to constantly be reminded about what I was talking about during conversations. I would walk into rooms of my house and stand there, wondering what I was there for. Telling this stuff to my doctor was a mistake, because she only thought I was crazy. My panicked attempts to figure things out and persistent scheduling only cemented this in her mind. She had decided that I was so crazy that I could manifest physical swelling, a loss of my period, and a weight gain of 30 pounds.

"Stress, likely Depression," she decided. "I am going to prescribe an anti-depressant to help you" she said.

I snapped "Do you know me!?!" "I am depressed *now* because I am gaining all of this weight and I'm f*cking lost inside of my own head, I can't wear shoes or stay awake and yes, *that* is stressful!" and then, ever so politely, I said "I hope you get strangled by a stethoscope." Exit, stage right.

The next doctor I saw was hell-bent on getting to the "bottom of it," and after examining my blood work, he asked me to come in immediately. I was told that my hemoglobin was so low I needed a transfusion, and I needed to begin eating red meat and taking ferrous sulfate and to eat more because I was basically dying of malnutrition. It appeared to him that my body has just "quit taking in nutrients" from my food. Shaking his head this internal medicine doc told me, "Your last doctor was an idiot." He got no argument there.

A couple months later, I still hadn't seen any major improvement in my condition. He told me to eat more red meat, spinach, kale, and fish. I told him that I had been eating those foods daily - but for some reason he didn't believe me, and told me that if I had been eating those foods I'd have surely gotten much better. My roommate at the time, Roxanne, vouched for me that those were, indeed, the foods that I had been eating. He told me to eat more. R

ealizing that the doctors were missing something and my condition progressively worsened, my mother Kimberly asked my dad for help in figuring out what was wrong with me. Looking for an answer, my father stumbled upon Celiac's Disease and suggested that I get tested for it. So, at my very next doctor's visit, I asked for the blood test.

My doctor said, and I quote, "You don't have Celiac's Disease. It's a rare, wasting disease. You on the other hand, are gaining weight. That's *not* it." I said "Give me the damn test!" A few weeks later the results were in. I got a phone call with the parting words of "Don't eat wheat."

Kimberly and I tried the paleo diet before, and I was not at all strict, even though I had seen her remarkable results. I still ate whole wheat bread and pasta, oatmeal and corn, rice and quinoa, and didn't take the diet too seriously. But after my diagnosis, within 8 days of a strict paleo diet, my legs turned pinker, my skin wasn't so gray, it didn't hurt to touch my skin, and I started sleeping 10 hours as opposed to 20. Within a month I felt like I had finally started making a real recovery. The swelling was down, the fog had lifted, and the weight had started to come off! Yay, me! Yay, Paleo!

But then I did something incredibly stupid. As an optimist, I truly believed that with "mind over matter" I could go to France with some friends from school and eat whatever I wanted to while I was there. I thought "Hey, I'm on vacation! I do what I want!" Unfortunately, I became incredibly ill again and my "mind over matter" experiment didn't work. I gained every bit of weight back (plus some) within the space of 2 weeks, and had been in more pain than I had ever been before. Upon my return, my family was horrified by my "Stay Pufft" appearance, so I went back to my strict paleo diet, and GI function returned after being at a painful standstill for weeks. But my body didn't bounce back and return to normal this time.

I began noticing sensitivities to everything that I ate. It was not just wheat, and not just grains, and not just soy or dairy that I was sensitive to – meat was making me sick. The Organic Chicken made me sick, the Organic Turkey made me sick, and God forbid I ate bacon! I thought I was going to die. My last hope, the so called "grass-fed" beef was also making me incredibly ill. The random stabbing pains and swelling returned with a vengeance and I hadn't even touched wheat in months. I was afraid I was going to lose my mind. I couldn't believe I wasn't getting better, or what I had done to myself in exchange for a croissant.

Although this explains some of my gruesome medical history, it doesn't explain how I came to care about food, food politics, farm animals, or sustainability. But there is one particular moment, however, that does.

It was when I was grocery shopping with my mother at a Whole Foods, standing in front of the meat counter. Scanning over the chicken, turkey, pork, lamb, and then the beef, I turned to Kimberly and remarked, "This doesn't make any sense whatsoever. The very thing that is supposed to be making me better is making me sick. Is it even possible to be allergic to everything?"

So I asked the butcher if the grass-fed labeled beef was indeed grass-fed, explaining that I was having somewhat of a reaction to it. He explained that it *was grass-fed,* but then it was grain finished for the last three months so it could get the proper nutrition before it went to the market, and "just eating grass isn't enough for them to be healthy." And then I realized, scanning over the meat counter again, that everything that I was eating was corn and soy-fed, all the way down to the farmed salmon. My head exploded.

It dawned on me that animals that were fed a species-appropriate diet, a paleo diet for the animals in other words, would make me better. My hypothesis was right, eating an animal that doesn't eat its species-appropriate and sustainable diet makes me sick, but eating those that do, saved my life again. I now have regular menses, and if I wanted to have a baby, I could. Looking at me, you would never know how sick and diseased and close to losing life and limbs I had been. And ever since, I have been interested in food, food politics, farm animals, and sustainability.

For the past 3 years, I have been actively promoting a Paleo Diet not only for myself, but for the animals we eat as well. A species-appropriate diet. My road to Paleo discovery can be seen more fully in my book, *Eat Paleo Save the World! Sustainability from an Omnivore's Perspective*, but also in the work I do with The Paleo Foundation, a non-profit organization that certifies paleo food and funds research and outreach programs for the explicit goal of advancing the Paleo Movement, which I founded as well.

To whom much is given, much is expected, and Paleo saved my life. Please check out my book on Amazon if you want to know more about why we need to eat paleo to preserve our natural resources. Check out the foundation's website at www.thepaleofoundation.org. And also check out the International Paleo Movement Group on Facebook at http://is.gd/paleogroup .

MATT CRANDALL

GILFORD, NEW HAMPSHIRE

In February of 2011, we were flying to Mexico for a week's vacation in the sun. I was weeks away from turning 38, father of two excellent teenagers, and engaged to an amazing woman. However, even at 6'5" tall, I was carrying a lot of extra weight. I refused to weigh myself, but I was wearing 3XLT shirts that were a little tight and size 48 waist pants without a belt.

In Mexico, I had plenty of fun but also a few scares. I felt like I was going to die after climbing two flights of stairs. I slathered myself in sunblock, but still ended up burning in the bright Mexican sun. I also had a small attack of Gout that swelled my foot a little and ached for a few days. I am lucky it wasn't worse.

On the last day of our trip, I downloaded our digital photos to my laptop and started going through them. My smile faded as I realized that I was probably fatter than I had ever been. The weird thing was that I had been eating smaller portions for a few weeks before we came to Mexico, hoping to drop a few pounds. Me in a zip line harness looked like a bag of Jell-O wrapped in tight rubber bands.

On the way back from Mexico, at the airport, I downloaded an audiobook to my Droid. A strange selection for me, because I normally love fiction. It was Gary Taubes' *Why We Get Fat and What to Do About It*. I was surprised to find myself saying this because I am typically a skeptic, but in the few hours it took to listen to audiobook, my world view changed. I went home and relentlessly searched for more information, both dissenting and supportive studies. Having struggled with weight my entire life, I almost cried on more than one occasion at the thought that that it had taken me so long to learn that grains were so toxic.

I struggled because I love food, I freaking LOVE it. I taught myself to cook by reading and watching TV and experimenting. I even wrote my own cookbook for my friends and family! My favorites were baking bread, pizzas, pasta, and my famous Death's Head Muffins, made of brownie batter, cheesecake batter, and chocolate chip cookie batter. It's no wonder I got to be so fat.

Weighing in at 308 pounds, I suffered from a few conditions that I had always thought were "age-related", despite not even being 40 yet. As I said, I had Gout that caused my feet to swell at the knuckle of the big toe and feel like they would explode. I also suffered from nightly heartburn for which I drank Maalox like it was a milkshake. My snoring was renowned far and wide for being able to shake walls, when I wasn't struggling for breath from sleep apnea. Of course, that's when I wasn't suffering from insomnia. Which is funny, because I would almost always fall asleep for an hour after every meal. I had problems with my knees, one hip, and my back too. If I twisted any of them wrong, I would be in constant pain for days.

Taubes' book touches on the idea of eating a natural diet, rich in saturated fats. My research led me then to Mark Sisson, author of *The Primal Blueprint* and marksdailyapple.com. It also led me to the community site Reddit and the sub group r/paleo. With these resources, and the additional scientific information a geek like me requires, I was ready to start.

On March 3rd, 2011, I removed all grains, processed foods, and sugar from the diet of my entire family. I am the grocery-getter and head chef, so I pretty much have the control. Gone was our pasta rich lasagna! Instead, I removed the noodles and used thin slices of eggplant and zucchini instead. Before, we had enjoyed tacos and burgers. So, I still made them, but used lettuce wraps instead of shells or buns.

I found a local farm that sold only grass-fed beef. I bought as much as I could afford and used it often. I also taught myself how to cook organ meats in such a way that my family did not know what they were eating, just that it tasted good. I traded favors with a few hunters who then gifted me with a few bundles of wild game like moose, elk, venison, and even black bear!

There was surprisingly little kicking or screaming in the family. Soda was replaced by iced tea lightly sweetened with honey and full of fresh mint or iced chai with a little coconut milk and honey. However, even the honey was lessened and taken away little by little. I started making the kids and my fiancée lunches to take with them so that temptations at school would pale in comparison. Who wants chicken soy nuggets when you have meat-crust pizza in your lunch?

Over the next few weeks, my family changed. I dropped weight so fast, I was a little afraid. "Nobody loses 15 pounds in a week, " my fiancé had whispered, looking at the scale seriously. I was grinning like an idiot. I felt freaking awesome! I literally felt like gravity had lessened, like I was on another planet.

My kids were both in sports, so I gave them both white and sweet potatoes to help them keep up. There's something interesting when you tell your daughter that her lunch is grilled heart and she says, "Yes!".

The entire family had transformed after a few months. My son had shed his belly and love handles and had enormous energy. He also lost all of his acne suddenly when we cut the sugar and began eating liver! My fiancée dropped 38 pounds and my daughter lost 12. I was the biggest guy and the biggest loser at 84 pounds lost in total. We all looked great and felt wonderful.

In those first 8 months, I had one attack of Gout. This had been a monthly occurrence before my change. It happened when I indulged in a few beers with some family members at a funeral. Also, my snoring lessened with each pound I lost. My kids would get up early in the morning instead of sleeping until noon. When it got dark out, I felt myself ready to fall peacefully asleep. I was incapable of staying up too late, yet I rarely felt sleepy after meals. I

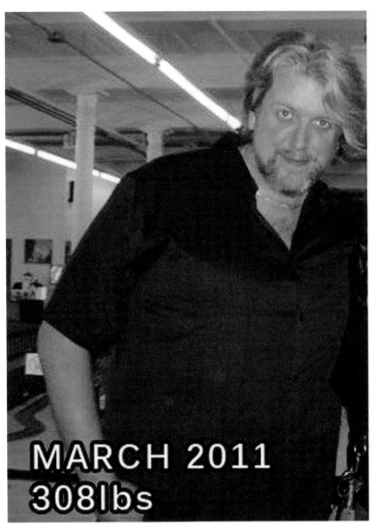

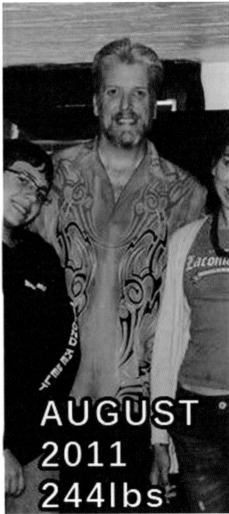

MARCH 2011
308lbs

AUGUST
2011
244lbs

also rarely felt hungry for 3 meals a day. What the heck was happening to me? I knew, and I liked it.

People I knew were amazed and sometimes wary. Many asked me what I was doing, while others said they thought maybe I was sick, except that I looked great. It's difficult to tell people about things that fly directly in the face of conventional wisdom or the "experts" in weight loss and health. When you feel the way I do, it's really hard not to try though. I am personally responsible for at least 12 Paleo converts outside of my own family. All of them are healthier, fitter, and happier than they were before.

After a few more months, I noticed I was fidgeting a lot. I would pace around the house and find things to do instead of lounging about watching TV. My whole family joined the gym down the road. I had been learning about the best workout for the kind of life we were living now. So, I made us up a heavy lifting, low cardio workout that could be done in 30-60 minutes, 3-4 times per week.

A year after I began this journey, I had a good friend say to me, "So, you're looking good now. When can you start to eat regular food again?"

I thought about the spaghetti dinners, the big sub sandwiches, and the packages of cookies and brownies and ice cream we used to buy weekly. None of it held any power over me anymore. My kids would still partake on special occasions, and each time they would say, "Why did I eat that.... it's not like it used to be."

I do admit that the one holiday season we have lived through while being Paleo, we cheated quite a bit. We ate things we shouldn't have for a week straight. We all felt like beaten dogs after that week was over. None of us complained about getting back on track either. It was a relief!

"I'm not ever going to eat the way I used to. I think this is forever!" I said. And the family agreed.

BRIAN COLLINS

BROOKLYN, NEW YORK

fitmedic68@yahoo.com , http://is.gd/fitmedic

June 2008 was a critical point in my life. Over the prior few years I had slowly been gaining weight, became less and less active, and started to experience physical problems. I had sleep apnea, my knees ached all the time, and I spent most of my time planning my next meal.

My family had expressed numerous times they were concerned about my weight and health - but I thought I was ok, or at least not as bad as people thought. But then I started having abdominal pains, and some shortness of breath while performing my job as a paramedic. So I finally caved in and went to a doctor.

After a battery of tests (EKG, stress test, upper/lower endoscopy, and blood work), I sat down with the doctor and the conversation went like this:

Doctor: "Ok so after looking at all the results, you are 40 years old, you weigh 267 pounds, you work all the time, eat poorly, don't exercise, don't do any drugs, and drink a little more than you should. You have an inflamed gallbladder and a fatty liver. You know what that makes you Brian?"

Me: "Ummmm…?"

Doctor: "It makes you a fat F&^&% of a human being!"

Me: "Wha…?!?"

Doctor: "Yep, so here's the deal. One of two things can happen. (1): You are a year away from diabetes and 2-3 years from a massive heart attack. You can keep going the way you are and I will prescribe all your meds, be there when they put the stents in your heart, and we can watch as your health deteriorates in front of you. Or (2): We can fix this.

Me: "I'm still here."

That's when I was able to get off my ass and start the work. Although he didn't know it then, he started me on the path to paleo eating. Eliminating dairy, white processed foods, and soda was the first step. And the weight gradually started coming off, at about a pound or so a week. And as long as I kept that up, I didn't have to take meds. I had been basically living on oatmeal, chicken, salads, rice, whole wheat pasta, and bread.

I started exercising, walking, and lifting weights as well as I could, and then I discovered Brazilian Jiu-Jitsu. Suffice to say, aside from eating paleo, this has been the most important change in my life, improving it in every facet. SO over the next two years I was losing weight and a fairly steady clip, but I still wasn't feeling a lot better. I felt sluggish and craved sweets constantly, but I thought I was getting better. My blood work improved some, and my doctor was happy. I went from seeing him once a month to once every three months, then once every six months.

I can't say for certain where I first read about paleo, but I think in a magazine article. So I went out and bought Loren Cordain, M.D.'s book *The Paleo Diet*. I was intrigued, but had many doubts. At the time I had started school to become a Registered Dietician, and Dr. Cordain's book defied what I was learning. I believed at least that diet was a huge part of health, and wanted to learn more. I delved on, and found Robb Wolf's and Mark Sisson's web pages very helpful. So I decided to try Robb's recommendation and go completely paleo for 30 days.

At first it was hard. Eating at work was a struggle because finding appropriate food is difficult when you are working overnights in the ambulance. I had to adapt to cooking a lot and bringing meals with me. Breakfast was very weird! I was eating chicken or tuna steak as my first meal of the day and it definitely took some getting used to. I craved pancakes and ice cream all the time. But the hardest part, hands down, was the reaction I was getting from friends. Most were horrified, saying I was undoing all the good I had achieved so far because I was eating so much meat and fat. By this point I had dropped about 50 pounds. Nobody believed that I could or would stay with it. But I did. Eating steak, and chicken on the bone, seafood of all kinds, and more vegetables then I had eaten the previous 42 years! And as I ate, I read and learned. I learned about whole clean foods, processed foods, and the health risks associated with them. It was one of the reasons that I left school - so I could focused on making myself more whole, as a healthy active human.

And the weight kept coming off! Breaking the 200 pound barrier was awesome! I also got my blue belt in jiu-jitsu. My energy level were at a higher level than I could ever remember, and I just felt younger. Avoiding the temptation of poor quality foods became easier. I found a couple of paleo groups on Facebook (http://is.gd/paleogroup) and on other websites. My recipes grew, and my confidence in what I was doing was solidified by meeting and learning from others who were doing paleo successfully.

My epiphany was at the end of the first 30 days, when I truly understood that this was not a "diet," but rather a complete lifestyle change. I have to admit that for maybe the first time in my life, I'm happy with the way I look. I've discovered a new confidence that had been

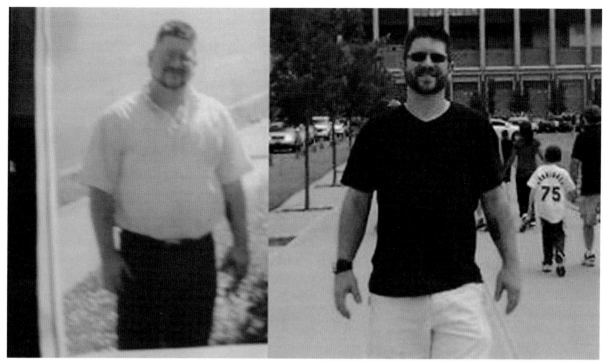

missing.

I write this four years after I started this journey, with two years paleo under by belt. I'm at a comfortable 178 pounds. My sleep apnea, fatty liver, inflamed gallbladder are all gone. I was able to keep myself off of medications that I believe in the long run would have only made things worse for me - and I may well be in the best shape of my life. I practice jiu-jitsu 3-4 times a week, lift twice a week, and alternate between short distance runs and sprints 2-3 times a week. I've also added yoga to my regular routine for flexibility.

My family has been incredibly supportive, some even adopting some of my paleo habits, and my friends are grudgingly acknowledging paleo's benefits. I keep getting more and more questions about the paleo approach to eating and lifestyle. Paying it forward can be the best way to acknowledge the people that helped you. So I became a personal trainer, and a Certified Sports Nutritionist and started my own business: FitMedic Training & Nutrition (http://is.gd/fitmedic). I am planning on making this my new career to help people who were in my situation reclaim their health and educate themselves to become the vital humans they can be. One of the most rewarding moments was when I walked into my doctor's office with my business cards. He smiled and said, "Nice work you skinny F@#&. "

TARA CHAPUT

RED DEER, ALBERTA, CANADA

March 2010: I turned 30 years old just 9 days after my 5th child was born. A year prior, I had decided that it was time to get serious about my health and my goal was to become a skinny, hot mama by the time I was 30. I had carried an extra 5-10 pounds from each pregnancy so by the time I decided to put my plan in action, I was 155 pounds. I was working out 2-3 times a week while eating clean and counting calories. The scale never moved and I was exhausted all of the time. The exhaustion was always blamed on something; the anemia during my 4th pregnancy, the 4 kids in 7 years, the bad sleep, the early mornings.

May 2010: At exactly 6 weeks postpartum, I was back in the gym and weighed 162 pounds. I tried very hard to juggle the hectic schedule that 5 kids bring but I still only managed to work out twice a week. At 3 months postpartum, I had reached my pre-pregnancy weight which was a first! The scale just stopped there though. I counted calories, often restricting the additional calories necessary during breastfeeding. I really didn't enjoy eating at all because I was eating the same foods, day in and day out. Oatmeal or egg white omelet for breakfast, salad for lunch, chicken breast and greens for supper. Snacks were 100 calorie snack packs, a weighed out portion of nuts or cheese, or a piece of fruit.

6 months postpartum, still no movement on the scale, and I was now also facing a medical issue that completely prevented me from working out. My life felt like it was spiraling out of control and I had no idea how to overcome even the simplest challenge. Over the next 6 months, I would bounce from high to low; defying doctor's orders and doing high intensity workouts only to see a rapid decline in my condition and resorting to a couch-bound sob fest. During my lows, I was eating whatever I wanted with no regard to calories/fat/sugar and I was having several anxiety/stress attacks every day.

Although I would claim that I was not depressed, my rock bottom moment found me in the middle of my kitchen floor, sobbing. My husband crouched beside me to hug me and I revealed to him that I wanted to drive into oncoming traffic. The only thing that kept me from doing that was the kids being in the vehicle with me.

It took another couple of months before I had a moment of real clarity. Friday nights were homemade pizza night and, because my husband was away, I ate 7 pieces. Within an hour, I was experiencing intense abdominal pain that left me completely incapable of moving. I had a hot bath with the hopes of the pain disappearing and by morning, the pain had mostly subsided. But the aches lasted for a couple of days more. A friend of mine had recently discovered that she had a gluten sensitivity, and she guided me through eliminating gluten from my diet. I replaced all of my food with gluten-free alternatives that tasted like corn starch and still, the scale didn't go down.

It was on a message board that I was introduced to Mark's Daily Apple and the paleo lifestyle. One of the articles that caught my eye on Mark's site discussed diet and depression. By then I had clued in to the fact that I was battling some pretty serious depression. A few ladies on the message board were getting ready to do a 30 day paleo challenge and, since gluten was already eliminated from my diet, I thought it might be a great idea to commit to 30 days.

May 2011: I was 31 and weighed 156 pounds. I threw myself into the paleo lifestyle head first and experienced 3 days worth of withdrawals. In just 2 weeks of doing it, I had to go buy new clothes because nothing fit! I even stuck to the 30 day challenge when we had to go away on vacation for 5 days because I was so happy with how quickly I was losing weight! But the weight loss really paled in comparison to the way I felt. For the first time in years, I felt clear

-minded. The day that it happened, it felt like a light switch just turned on. I didn't have to force a fake smile because I was genuinely happy! I didn't need to nap during the day because I felt energized! I didn't imagine running away from home because I was no longer overwhelmed by my life! After the 30 days, I had seen enough changes (physical and mental) that I knew I couldn't go back. 6 weeks into the paleo lifestyle, I lost 15 pounds and I asked my husband to make the switch too. 3 months in, I felt confident enough to switch all 5 kids and we saw almost immediate positive changes in all of them.

May 2012: I was 32 and weighed 125 pounds. I lost 30 pounds and my husband lost almost 40 pounds in one year - and we have gained a lot, just not weight, lol. I have overcome a depression that I'm sure would have eventually cost me my marriage, my family, and possibly my life. I have overcome years of mysterious stomach pains. I have taken control of my life and that has been the best part of this lifestyle change.

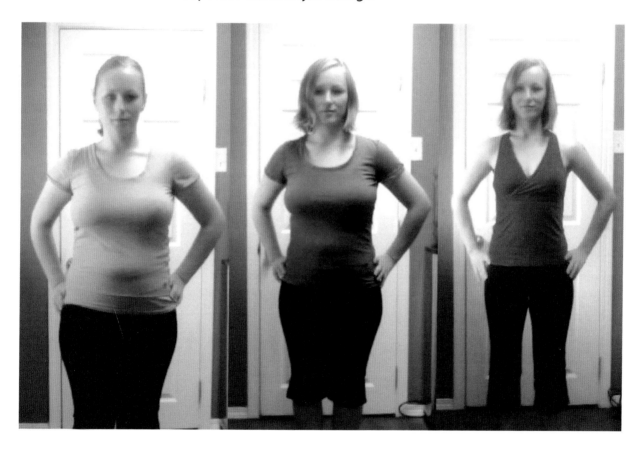

I enjoy sharing the passion I used to have for food with the kids again. Food isn't the enemy or the source of my guilt anymore; it's an outlet for my creativity. Our meals are typically very simple…quality protein, fat, and lots of vegetables. We love trying new foods and the kids have eaten things that I never could have imagined! Discovering that there is a connection between quality food and health has given me the motivation I need to pursue a degree in natural nutrition. When I enrolled, my goal was to lead even a single person into a healthier lifestyle. Then I realized that I have led the most important person there already: Myself.

TESS

FREMONT, CALIFORNIA

July 2005 – the start of my rapid health decline
Age: 21, weight 160 pounds

Started having health problems (chronic urticaria and angioedema, extreme exhaustion, GI cramps so bad that I couldn't get out of bed for days, diarrhea with undigested food, acne)

Typical meals (vegetarian): cheese pizza, veggie burger on whole-wheat bun with cheese and fries, macaroni and cheese

May 2007 – lost weight with South Beach diet, but health problems continued
Age: 23, weight 140 pounds

Typical meals (South Beach): turkey lunchmeat wrapped in lettuce with low fat string cheese, salad with plain chicken & small amounts of whole-wheat bread

January 2009 – body and mind falling apart
Age: 25, 140 pounds

My health problems had been rapidly getting worse, and by January of 2009 I was completely falling apart. I was still having chronic urticaria and angioedema, acne, and no energy, and had added daily migraines, daily stomachache, and chronic heartburn to my list of symptoms. I could barely get out of bed, was having trouble thinking, and my brain seemed to just space out.

Attempted solutions:
GI doctor: diagnosed IBS, prescribed anti-depressant, Zantac, Zyrtec, Bentyl
Neurologist: found no issues on EEG or MRI, no ideas
General: trying to eat healthy, too exhausted to exercise, sleeping ~20 hours a day

February 10, 2009 – found my miracle
Age 25, 140 pounds

I will never forget February 10, 2009. I woke up in the middle of the night and felt like I wasn't in my body anymore. My mind started trying to make sense out of it. Am I dreaming? Am I dead? I moved my arms and legs, touched my face. I was there, lying in my bed, but all of my senses seemed different. I couldn't feel any pain in my body. I had forgotten what it was like to not have a headache, stomachache, or pain in my muscles and joints. I had gotten so used to 24-7 pain that it had become how I interacted with the world and how I recognized my presence in my body. Lying in my bed, I just felt peace. Then I noticed that my brain seemed to be working again. I started thinking of all of the signs of illness throughout my life and realized that I hadn't actually felt this good since I was a kid, probably ~12 years old.

I fell back asleep, and then woke up at 6:30am. I was completely awake with tons of energy. I jumped out of bed and ran downstairs. My boyfriend was sitting in our living room, and when he saw me bound down the stairs with a huge smile on my face, his jaw hit the floor. It was probably the first time in our 3-year relationship that he had seen me wake up that early, and the most energetic he had EVER seen me.

What was my solution? Giving up gluten. On February 7, 2009, I had talked to my mom on the phone. I was desperate. I thought that I was dying, and asked my mom if she knew of any genetic conditions in my family. I asked her to to tell me anything that came to mind. One of the things she said was that my grandma "couldn't eat wheat." I had heard of celiac disease, and it had crossed my mind during my years of declining health, but I had brushed it off because I thought that people with celiac were supposed to be skinny. This time I didn't brush it off, though. After I got off the phone with my mom, I went online to search for the symptoms of celiac disease. I looked at the list of symptoms and started crossing off all of the ones that I had had. I read that Finland and Ireland have some of the highest incidents of the disease in the world (my mom's ancestors had moved to the US from Finland just 2 generations earlier, and most of my dad's ancestors had moved from Ireland 2-3 generations before). What first sounded like a long shot was beginning to sound more plausible. I stopped searching and decided that I was going to start eating gluten free right then. Three days later, I realized that it was the best decision I had ever made in my life.

My journey since February 10, 2009 has not been easy, but I will never go back. I have had my setbacks along the way, learning how sensitive I am to gluten and that there were other foods that my body felt better without. I first learned that my body wasn't responding well to dairy.

I started to experiment and then I came across the next level of health.

May 2011 to present – health upgrade: PALEO
Age 26-28
weight: 130-140 pounds

I had come across blogs talking about the paleo diet when I was looking for gluten and dairy free recipes. I was a scientist and thinking about the evolutionary framework for diet was appealing. Everything that I was reading seemed to make sense, and I relished the idea personally - it made me stop thinking that I was a "broken person" with celiac, because it was expected that many people wouldn't be completely adapted to grains. I read blogs, books, and listened to podcasts for almost a year (starting in 2010) before I proclaimed, "this makes sense. I'm going to really try this 100%." It wasn't too much of a transition for me to go 100%. I just took out the little bit of quinoa, rice, and beans that I was eating, and I continued to feel better.

For the past three years, I have not had any migraines like I used to get. I have tons of energy, and started running races (up to a half marathon) and doing triathlons. I have not had any urticaria or angioedema. I haven't had any moments of my brain spacing out, and only get the dizziness/off balance feelings when I accidentally eat some gluten. I have had some setbacks along the way, feeling frustrated that I have to pay so much attention to the food I'm

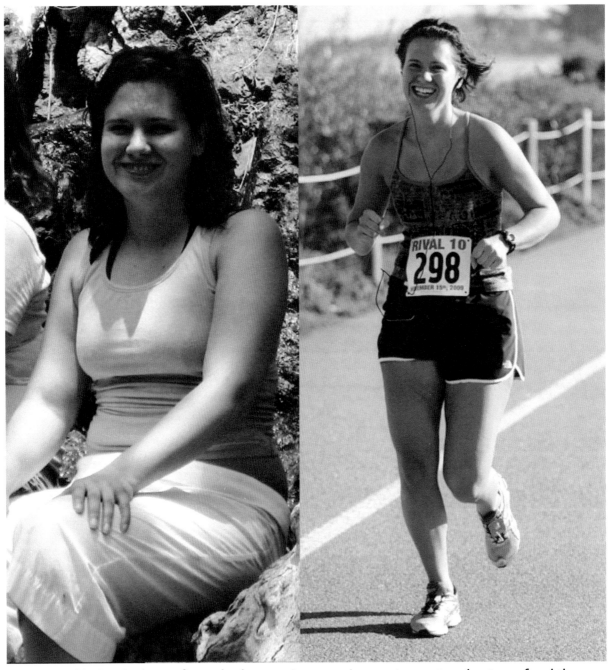

eating, and being jealous of people that can just stop in a restaurant and eat any food they want. A few times I have rebelled and said "screw it. I am just going to eat junk food!" It feels exhilarating while I'm doing it, but then I feel like crap. Eventually I will learn.

My family is happy that I am healthy now, and some of them have even gone gluten free themselves. My boyfriend (who saw me the morning that I found my miracle) is now my husband, and is supportive. When we eat out at restaurants, he pushes the staff to make sure that I don't get contaminated, and our kitchen is almost gluten free. He told me that it makes our lives harder that I have to be so careful about my diet, but that he recognizes that because of it we eat healthier and he will end up better off.

Typical meals: shrimp and veggie omelet, salad with scallops, grass-fed roast with carrots and root vegetables.

BRIAN OTTO

NESBIT, MISSISSIPPI

xanderelectric@comcast.net

In June of 2006 I turned 30 years old. My first (and only) child was due in September. I am a Firefighter – and I considered myself to be fit. My beautiful wife of ten years, Ally, happens to be a vegetarian. At thirty weeks she was suddenly diagnosed with preeclampsia. I had no idea what that was. Ignorance is bliss, or was it?   Our "healthy" diets were certainly failing us. Our newborn daughter Xander, was premature but fortunately healthy.   Ally was on blood pressure medicine for months after Xander was born and was unable to breast feed because of it. Xander was put on Nutramigen (the Filet Mignon of Formula, with a price tag to match). I decided to do some research. I was shocked to learn that all of the conventional wisdom of the American diet (low fat, high grains, vegetable oils) was anything but healthy. This was confirmed again and again, after a lengthy discussion with our pediatrician, OBGYN and family physician.

Ally had "baby weight" to lose.   I had "sympathy weight" to lose. Who among us hasn't tried cutting calories and increasing exercise? This is difficult enough normally, but when you are new parents, it is almost impossible. Add sleep deprivation to busy work schedules and sleep takes priority over exercise every time. It's not that I didn't have good intentions of going to the gym - I did. But intentions don't get results. You tell yourself that working is going to combat that calorie-loaded casserole dish some sweet lady brought you for dinner last night, along with dessert to match. My Wife calls them "push presents" I call them kryptonite.   At six feet tall, I weighed 203 pounds. It seemed normal to me because I live in Mississippi (the fattest of our fifty states), and because I was raised the American way, on fast food like everyone else. If you are what you eat, I was fast cheap and easy. However, when you have a hot wife and a beautiful baby girl, the last thing you want to be is an embarrassment. And when you're mostly fat and have no muscle definition, it's not sexy.

It was March 2007, and my Ultimate Goal was almost unattainable. I had always wanted to be in the elite: A Mississippi State Certified Smoke Diver. It's very physical and very hard; some say it's the Navy Seal of Firefighting. Certification consists of five days of hell spent at the State Fire Academy, away from your family, testing your physical and mental limitations while watching your "brothers" leaving in ambulances because they "didn't measure up." I made it! I measured up, barely. I had to admit to myself just how un-fit I actually was. I got home and got into a zone. No really, I read The Zone. The Zone Diet was very challenging. I saw some physical results, but at the end of day it was still a "diet."

Then my Lieutenant opened a crossfit gym, and I began doing these very unusual work outs at the fire station with him. I started to see some real results.

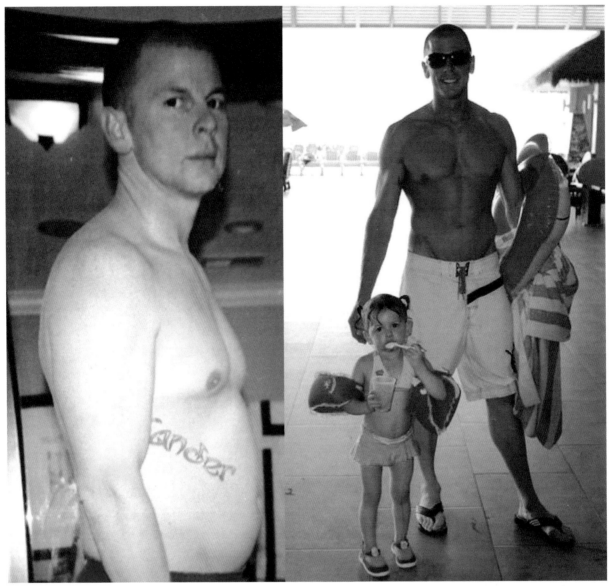

It was then that I was introduced to a term that would change my life. Paleo. Eating paleo is eating like our ancestors - only what you can hunt or gather. Sounds simple enough, but practicing this in a modern world is harder than you would think. I started experimenting, (paleo scientist that I am) first with exercise then with food. I started doing more weight lifting and lower intensity training. I began to notice the effects food had on me and how they made me feel. For the first time since early childhood, I no longer needed a prescription for acid reflux. Then I read *The Primal Blueprint* by Mark Sisson and *The Paleo Solution* by Robb Wolf. I became obsessed reading anything paleo related. I learned among many things that food is a drug, very addictive (and I was an addict). Now, I'm a member of the modern world. I don't gather or hunt (my wife's vegetarian, but not the kind that wears plastic shoes). So what's a modern day caveman to do? Cut out all man made processed foods. Anything that did not exist back then, it really is that simple. If you didn't kill or grow it, don't eat it. This includes grains, which are processed to be edible by humans.

It is now 2012, and I am still six feet tall but only 165 pounds and just 5% body fat. According to my research, this should work equally as well for everyone else; just as it worked for cavemen for over 100,000 years. I made a decision to help as many people achieve health (God Willing) as I possibly can.

We all have goals, whether it is losing weight, gaining lean muscle, or just being in good health. The most important thing to remember is that they are attainable for everyone. And you don't have to do it alone: this book will assist you in your journey. As well as I hope, inspire you to be your own personal best. I believe in a healthy mind, body and spirit. I haven't looked back, and I have no regrets. I only wish I had discovered paleo sooner.

RICH KRZYZANOWSKI

CHICAGO, ILLINOIS

chykynlyps@gmail.com , www.naturalevo.com

My transformation journey starts in August of 2010. I was 28. I stood 6', 2" and weighed 240 pounds. I was sick. I was sick of being sick. I had no self-confidence. I had heartburn all the time. I was eating over-the-counter antacids like they were candy. I had trouble sleeping regularly. I hate doctors, so I refused to see them because their only tools are poisonous prescription medications. I rarely worked out because I would be in so much pain afterward. I hated myself and my life, and I was doing nothing to correct it.

By a stroke of luck, my little sister started practicing yoga and invited me to join her. I was a bit skeptical, but I went anyway. I was hooked. I felt good after yoga. I started to see some results, slowly. I was sleeping a little bit better and losing some weight, but I was still trying to follow a low-fat, high-carb diet. I started practicing yoga six days a week, but something still wasn't exactly right. If I was working so hard, why was I stuck with belly fat? And where were my six-pack abs? I had lost about 30 pounds and I was certainly feeling better about myself, but I knew that there was a piece of the puzzle that was missing. That piece was a proper diet.

My dear friend introduced me to paleo in the fall of 2011. I looked at it and instantly knew that I had to give it a shot! For one reason or another, I put off starting it until January 1, 2012. If I knew then what I know now, I wouldn't have waited another second. I did a Whole 30 (a specific paleo protocol challenge) for the month of January. And it was eye-opening, to say the least. At first, I had trouble cutting out the sugar. I have always had a sweet tooth, but once I got over the first few days of carb flu/withdrawal (headaches, body aches, trouble sleeping), I felt amazing. I had so much energy, I felt like I didn't need sleep. And when it was time to sleep, I slept better than I had been in a VERY long time. I ate when I was hungry, and sometimes, that was only once a day!!!

As I progressed through that first month, I knew my body was changing. I had been stuck at 210 pounds for so long; I was convinced that my body had found its happy weight. By the end of January, I was down to 195 pounds and I was starting to see definition in places that I had never seen it before! My lower abs were finally starting to poke through the layer of fat that had always covered them. And I was getting stronger. I have always been pretty strong, but once I started paleo I could feel the difference in my yoga practice. I could hold my arm balances longer and more steadily than I could before. I was not getting fatigued. I was recovering much more quickly. Back when I was eating grains, breads, and pastas, I always felt like I was swollen. I used to get a sort of mental fog after I ate, and I would feel the need to take a nap. I could actually feel my blood pressure rise after meals. My fingers would swell up. I would feel dehydrated a lot.

My typical meal was something you might find recommended by the USDA. I was just always under the impression that humans were supposed to feel like crap after eating.

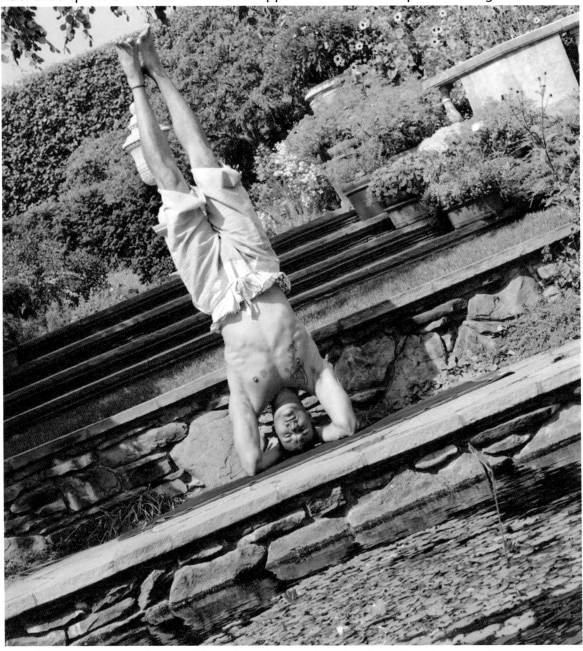

Now, my diet consists of tons of fat! I love fats, and my body responds so well to the energy that they provide me. I eat grass-fed or pastured animals. Beef is my favorite. But bacon is

REALLY my favorite. Sometimes (okay, usually), when I make bacon, I will let the fat congeal at the bottom of the pan and then scoop it out with my finger for a snack. Bacon does a body good! Believe it! I tend to eat whatever organic vegetables are available at the farmers' market. My plate now looks about 70% covered with meat and 30% covered in vegetables. If I have roasted vegetables, I will give myself a nice, hearty dollop of butter or bacon grease or beef tallow on the side.

Before starting yoga, my mental clarity was about 3 out of 10. Once I had been practicing yoga for a year, I thought it was an 11. But once I went paleo, my mental clarity has been about 20 out of 10. It blows me away. Now when I eat, I feel energized and ready to face whatever challenges might come my way. I even feel less stressed. I'm not saying that I have less stress in my life, but I am saying that the stress I do feel is more easily managed because my body is no longer working so hard to fight off a crap diet. It allows me to focus on taking care of my mental, emotional, and spiritual states. I have noticed that the amount of fat that I eat has an effect on my mental state. If I haven't had enough fat, I get tense and feel like I'm stressed out and not able to deal with it very well. A few spoons of butter or bacon grease will usually clear that right up.

As I am right now, I feel better than I ever have before. I look better than I ever have before, and it gives me more confidence. I'm 30 years old. I'm still 6', 2", but now I weigh 185 pounds. I have more muscular definition that I have ever had. That excites the hell out of me! I love being able to see my abs!

Paleo has certainly come with some challenges. It has been difficult in finding acceptance from my family in some regards. The toughest part is when we are all sitting down for a meal and people are passing the bread basket around. I usually say, "No, thanks. I'll just have butter." Inevitably, someone will make a snide comment about my diet. It is very difficult for me not to say "Enjoy your systemic inflammation and lifestyle diseases!" because, at the end of the day, they are family. It is tough to be healthy amongst a group of people that I care about and want to help, but who won't accept my help because they have grown up with popular misconceptions about saturated fat.

I no longer have any issues with heartburn. I haven't taken an antacid in the nine months since I have been paleo. I sleep like a baby whenever I want to. I just feel great all the time! Thank you paleo!

TIM SWART, A.K.A. DR. BACON

CANYON COUNTRY, CALIFORNIA

www.allinpaleo.com , www.facebook.com/allinpaleo , allinpaleo@gmail.com

I started paleo on April 28, 2011, at the age of 42, with a weight of 312.8 pounds. My overall health was poor and deteriorating. I was a type II diabetic with joint issues, inflammation, headaches, and serious obesity. I was taking 1000 mg Metformin twice a day, and 45mg Actos once a day. My feet cracked and bled, and any time I trimmed my nails, or had any cuts on my feet or with my toenails, I would get a staph infection – up to 4 times a year - which caused me to be on multiple antibiotics, and pain medication. I took up to 3000mg of Advil/Motrin/ Ibuprofen daily just to deal with the pain.

Back when I was first diagnosed, I took it really hard, but followed what the doctor said; watch what I eat, eat a high carb, high fiber, low fat diet, minimize red meat, and fatty meats, eat more fruits and vegetables. I went to the gym 2 or 3 times a week, and like every other time I "dieted", it just wasn't working.

I saw my doctor several times a year, I had to have surgery on my 2nd toe on my right foot in 2009. It took a long time to heal due to the diabetes. After a while, I wouldn't heal like I used to, and I got my last bad staph infection - they said it was MRSA – and in August 2010, I ended up in the hospital where they had to open and drain the wound, and I was on IV antibiotics for 8 hours.

That open wound took 5 months to heal. I saw my doctor in November of 2010, and he wanted me on insulin because the drugs obviously were not bringing my sugars down. I told him "no thank you, I refuse to be on insulin." That is the last time I have been to the doctor.

I knew I had to find a way to beat this thing.

I was working a very stressful job that I had been at for 15 years when I discovered Paleo. I was working 6 days a week, every weekend, on call 24/7, not sleeping well at all (3-4 hours a night most days). On April 27, 2011, I was working from home, just listening to conference calls. I was on my computer and searched Holistic Diabetes Cures and an article from Mark Sisson at Mark's Daily Apple popped up in the search results. http://marksdailyapple.com/ diabetes. I clicked on that link and my life was changed…FOREVER!!

I read, and read, and clicked on link after link, and was introduced to the paleo way of eating. It totally made sense to me. I had been on every diet there was except being a vegetarian/ vegan because I could NEVER give up meat, and at first paleo reminded me of the Atkins diet. I had done well on Atkins about 10 years earlier, and thinking back on it: Had I stuck with Atkins, I probably would never have gotten diabetes.

But I digress. Back to reading, and reading. That day I spent about 8 hours reading everything I could about this "diet." I decided right then and there that I would start the next day. And I did. April 28, 2011 is my paleo birthday.

Needless to say my paleo instincts were to go back to my prior experience, Atkins style, eating very low carb (it just made sense for diabetics to not eat carbs - the thing that causes spikes in sugar) instead of what we were told to eat. It was no wonder that it hadn't worked. I had no problem eating meats, fats, cheese, veggies and nuts. I decided to cut the sugar/carby stuff out and see what happened. I was eating eggs and bacon for breakfast before work. I would bring meat and spinach/arugula/nuts to make a salad. I made my own salsa for dressing, and dinner would be meat and a veggie. Like all "new diets" I saw results rather quickly, with my weight dropping 17 pounds in the first 30 days!!

AWESOMESAUCE!

But here's the real awesome part of my first month: On day 1 my fasting blood glucose was 190. That was the reading I got on the morning of April 28, 2011. Well after 2 weeks paleo, my fasting BG was now 140!!! A 50 point drop in 2 weeks eating like a caveman!! Say what??!!

At the time I started having some "bathroom" issues, and after reading and reading, I never stopped reading about paleo, I decided to QUIT MY DIABETES DRUGS!! The side effect of the drugs was diarrhea, and that's what I was experiencing. It was a huge leap to take, but I was feeling awesome, and many days I'd even forget to take them, so what the hell...well the following 2 weeks the weight kept coming off, and on day 30 my fasting blood glucose reading WAS 125!!!!!!! A 65 point drop in one freaking month!! Are you kidding me?!?! I had found the answer!

I dropped 33 pounds in the first 3 months, without hardly any exercise. I realized that I needed to dedicate my life to this lifestyle. I decided to quit my stressful job, and do whatever I could to help others live and beat this disease of diabetes!! I had heard about this new exercise called "CrossFit" and I searched to see if I had a gym in my area. Luckily we did. I decided that I would go check it out to see what it was all about.

Well, as most people who try CrossFit will tell you, it's addicting. And yes I got addicted. I started on my 43rd birthday July 26, 2011, and I had never experienced workouts like that in my life. I was energized. It was good, quick, challenging, and everything can be scaled to your ability. I have great coaches and have made a ton of friends for life being part of the CrossFit family!

I the first seven months, I lost a total of 50 pounds, and my fasting BG numbers were routinely in the 100 and mid 90's range now!! I was basically normal with my readings…and I was totally hooked on THIS LIFESTYLE!!

The 8th month started my plateau, it was now December, and I had dropped another 5 pounds through December 17, 2011. I went to a Christmas party and had a few drinks, a few "treats" (non-paleo). I tried to find ways to make my favorite holiday items acceptable, and I ate them with no thought...I gained 4 pounds total from November to December. So began the tweaking and trying different things, to get the fires burning again. I gained and lost the same 10 pounds for months.

At my 1 year anniversary on April 28, 2012, I took my BG reading for my big 1 year post, and I had achieved a number I had never seen before!!!! 83!!! I WAS SHOCKED!! My weight was 55 pounds down, at 257.8 pounds. I took photos and the transformation, while still in progress, was nothing short of amazing. In one year, I had dropped 14.1% body fat, dropped 34.5 inches, and I went from 3/4XL shirts to 2X, from 42 inch size pants to 36 inch. I had not been in 36 inch pants since I was a teenager. I will always be a large man (I am 6'4" and have very wide shoulders), so I don't expect my shirt size to change too much. But as I continue to

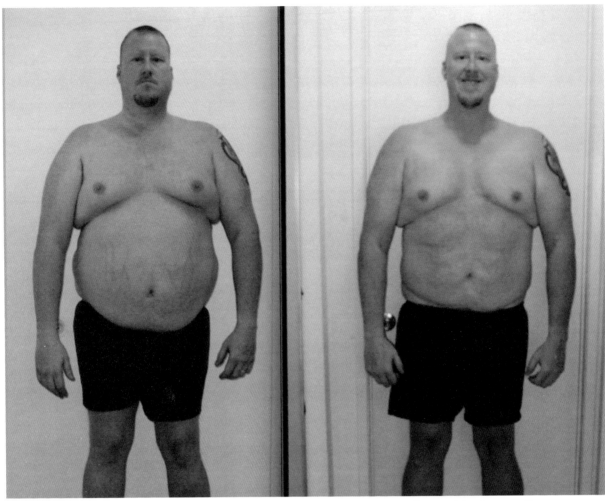

evolve and tweak my eating, I know that I'll drop the remaining fat and be in smaller pants some day.

My diabetes was gone, my inflammation was gone, and no more medications!! I am not in pain anymore (except after a great workout) and that just lets me know that I'm working my body!! My sleep has improved too, and I wake up every morning without an alarm as soon as it is light outside.

I have yet to go back to the doctor. I really have no need to other than curiosity. But I really am so laid back now and I know internally I'm the healthiest I've been in my entire life. Some day I will, and that will be when I hit my goal weight.

I have dedicated my life to this lifestyle and have interacted with THOUSANDS of people through Facebook and meeting in person through my Facebook page, and through groups like the IPMG (International Paleo Movement Group, http://is.gd/paleogroup), the largest paleo group on Facebook, which I help administer. I have posted my progress on my blog, and Facebook page, and I am working with some very important people in the Paleo community on a project that will be life changing for many. I am ALL IN with this lifestyle!!